Swing Beds

Brookings Dialogues on Public Policy

The presentations and discussions at Brookings conferences and seminars often deserve wide circulation as contributions to public understanding of issues of national importance. The Brookings Dialogues on Public Policy series is intended to make such statements and commentary available to a broad and general audience, usually in summary form. The series supplements the Institution's research publications by reflecting the contrasting, often lively, and sometimes conflicting views of elected and appointed government officials, other leaders in public and private life, and scholars. In keeping with their origin and purpose, the Dialogues are not subjected to the formal review procedures established for the Institution's research publications. Brookings publishes them in the belief that they are worthy of public consideration but does not assume responsibility for their accuracy or objectivity. And, as in all Brookings publications, the judgments, conclusions, and recommendations presented in the Dialogues should not be ascribed to the trustees, officers, or other staff members of the Brookings Institution.

Swing Beds

*Assessing Flexible Health Care
in Rural Communities*

Papers by JOSHUA M. WIENER

ANTHONY R. KOVNER & HILA RICHARDSON

STEVEN A. FINKLER

JOHN HOLAHAN

PETER W. SHAUGHNESSY

HELEN L. SMITS

BRUCE C. VLADECK

presented at a conference at the Brookings Institution,
February 24, 1986

Edited by JOSHUA M. WIENER

THE BROOKINGS INSTITUTION
Washington, D.C.

About Brookings

THE BROOKINGS INSTITUTION is a private nonprofit organization devoted to research, education, and publication in economics, government, foreign policy, and the social sciences generally. Its principal purpose is to bring knowledge to bear on the current and emerging public policy problems facing the American people. In its research, Brookings functions as an independent analyst and critic, committed to publishing its findings for the information of the public. In its conferences and other activities, it serves as a bridge between scholarship and public policy, bringing new knowledge to the attention of decisionmakers and affording scholars a better insight into policy issues. Its activities are carried out through three research programs (Economic Studies, Governmental Studies, Foreign Policy Studies), a Center for Public Policy Education, a Publications Program, and a Social Science Computation Center.

The Institution was incorporated in 1927 to merge the Institute for Government Research, founded in 1916 as the first private organization devoted to public policy issues at the national level; the Institute of Economics, established in 1922 to study economic problems; and the Robert Brookings Graduate School of Economics and Government, organized in 1924 as a pioneering experiment in training for public service. The consolidated institution was named in honor of Robert Somers Brookings (1850–1932), a St. Louis businessman whose leadership shaped the earlier organizations.

Brookings is financed largely by endowment and by the support of philanthropic foundations, corporations, and private individuals. Its funds are devoted to carrying out its own research and educational activities. It also undertakes some unclassified government contract studies, reserving the right to publish its findings.

A Board of Trustees is responsible for general supervision of the Institution, approval of fields of investigation, and safeguarding the independence of the Institution's work. The President is the chief administrative officer, responsible for formulating and coordinating policies, recommending projects, approving publications, and selecting the staff.

Editor's Preface

IN MANY rural communities there is both a surplus of hospital beds and a shortage of nursing home beds. At the same time, medicare and medicaid regulations generally require that acute care and long-term care be provided in physically separate facilities. One possible solution to this dilemma is to waive these regulations and allow small rural hospitals to use the same bed to provide either acute or long-term care, whichever is most needed. This concept, known as swing beds, has been implemented; it simultaneously increases the use of hospital facilities and reduces the need for transferring patients to distant nursing homes.

This volume in the series of Brookings Dialogues on Public Policy examines many issues related to swing beds, including cost effectiveness, reimbursement policy, the effect on access to nursing home care, and the quality of care. The papers were presented at a conference held at the Brookings Institution on February 24, 1986.

Anthony R. Kovner and Hila Richardson of the Rural Hospital Program of Extended-Care Services at New York University provided invaluable help in organizing the conference and critiquing the papers. Jeffrey Merrill and Saul Kilstein of the Robert Wood Johnson Foundation were instrumental in bringing this project to fruition. Nancy Davidson edited the manuscript for publication, and Sheila E. Murray and Diana L. Coupard provided research assistance.

The Brookings Institution is grateful to the Robert Wood Johnson Foundation for its support for the writing of the papers, the conference, and the production of this volume.

Joshua M. Wiener

January 1987
Washington, D.C.

Contents

Introduction and Summary

JOSHUA M. WIENER

HISTORICALLY, many hospitals, especially in rural areas, have provided both acute and long-term care in the same facility. However, current medicare and medicaid regulations require that hospitals provide long-term care in a "distinct-part" unit physically separate from their acute-care beds.[1]

Many small rural hospitals have trouble meeting this requirement because of the nature of their physical plant, limited accounting capabilities, and insufficient demand and skilled staff. At the same time, many of these hospitals have excess acute-care beds in communities where there is a scarcity of nursing home beds. Thus the swing-bed concept was introduced in order to allow small rural hospitals with fewer than fifty beds to use their beds interchangeably to provide either acute care or nursing home care, with reimbursement based on the specific type provided. Allowing the use of beds in this manner provides small hospitals with greater flexibility in meeting fluctuating demands for inpatient hospital and nursing home care.

History of the program   Statutory authority for the current medicare and medicaid swing-bed program was added to the Social Security Act by legislation passed in 1980.[2] Implementing regulations were issued by the Health Care Financing Administration on July 20, 1982.[3] As of July 1985, approximately 700 hospitals were participating in the swing-bed program. Participation has increased rapidly since the implementation of the medicare hospital prospective payment system. Under current law, when swing beds are used for acute-

---

1. A distinct-part unit must be a physically identifiable unit consisting of all the beds within that unit (such as a separate building, floor, wing, or corridor) and must meet health, safety, and additional requirements. The distinct part is reimbursed as a separate entity.

2. *Omnibus Reconciliation Act of 1980*, Conf. Rept. 96-1479, 96 Cong. 2 sess. (Government Printing Office, 1980), sec. 904, adding secs. 1883 and 1913 to the Social Security Act, which were later renumbered as 42 U.S.C. 1395tt and 42 U.S.C. 1396l (1985).

3. 47 Fed. Reg. 31518–33 (1982).

1

care services by medicare patients, the hospital receives the usual diagnosis-related group (DRG) payment per case; when patients are discharged into nursing home status, the hospital receives additional payments on a per diem basis. Thus hospitals with excess capacity receive more reimbursement under the swing-bed program.

The national program under which rural hospitals are currently providing swing-bed care is the outgrowth of a demonstration sponsored by the Health Care Financing Administration (HCFA) in the mid-1970s involving more than 100 rural hospitals in four states: Utah, Texas, Iowa, and South Dakota. The demonstration was exhaustively evaluated by Peter Shaughnessy and colleagues at the University of Colorado Center for Health Services Research.[4]

Since 1982 the Robert Wood Johnson Foundation has funded a national demonstration to promote the swing-bed concept by establishing models of how small rural hospitals with excess capacity can provide quality long-term care services in areas with nursing home shortages. The University of Colorado research team is currently evaluating the Robert Wood Johnson Foundation demonstration and the response of rural hospitals to the existing swing-bed law and regulatory requirements and to the incentives of the medicare hospital prospective payment system.[5]

Participation

The number of hospitals participating in the swing-bed program has grown rapidly, from 149 in December 1983 to 688 in July 1985, a 362 percent increase. Table 1 shows that thirteen states had twenty-three or more participating hospitals in July 1985: Arkansas, Colorado, Iowa, Kansas, Minnesota, Mississippi, Missouri, Montana, Nebraska, North Dakota, South Dakota, Texas, and Wisconsin.

Limits on Participation

Participation in the medicare and medicaid programs is limited to small rural hospitals with fewer than fifty inpatient hospital beds. The regulations count all inpatient hospital beds maintained

4. Peter W. Shaughnessy and others, *An Evaluation of Swing Bed Experiments to Provide Long-Term Care in Rural Hospitals*, vols. 1 and 2 (Denver: University of Colorado Center for Health Services Research, March 1980).

5. Peter W. Shaughnessy and others, *Hospital Swing Beds in the United States: Initial Findings* (Denver: University of Colorado Center for Health Services Research, November 1985).

Table 1. *Distribution of Certified Swing-Bed Hospitals, by State,
December 1983–July 1985*

State[a]	Number of hospitals					
	12/83	3/84	7/84	10/84	12/84	7/85
Alaska	1	1	1	2	2	6[b]
Arizona	0	4	6	6	6	6
Arkansas	1	1	5	8	16	25
California	3	3	4	5	6	6
Colorado	2	9	13	15	16	23[b]
Georgia	0	3	4	5	6	9
Hawaii	2	2	2	2	2	1[b]
Idaho	3	3	4	4	4	9[b]
Illinois	0	1	2	5	8	16
Indiana	1	1	2	2	2	4
Iowa	33	37	44	44[c]	86	92[d]
Kansas	7	10	16	16[c]	40	63[b]
Kentucky	1	0	1	1	1	1[b]
Louisiana	0	0	0	1	1	4
Minnesota	3	4	24	56	63	79
Mississippi	4	4	4	4	8	30[b]
Missouri	7	13	16	16[c]	32	44
Montana	9	13	17	19	20	26
Nebraska	5	3	5	5[c]	14	36[d]
Nevada	4	4	4	4	4	3[b]
New Hampshire	2	2	2	2	2	2
New Mexico	8	8	8	9	9	13[b]
North Carolina	1	4	7	7	7	8
North Dakota	14	20	20	21	21	29[b]
Ohio	0	0	0	2	2	2
Oklahoma	1	1	1	1	4	13
South Carolina	0	0	0	0	0	7
South Dakota	19	20	21	22	23	27[b]
Tennessee	0	1	1	3	3	7
Texas	2	2	4	8	17	26
Utah	7	7	7	8	8	10[b]
Vermont	0	0	0	0	0	1[b]
Washington	2	5	8	8	9	10[b]
Wisconsin	6	7	15	16	24	38
Wyoming	1	5	5	5	5	12[b]
Total	149	198	273	332	471	688

Source: Peter W. Shaughnessy and others, *Hospital Swing Beds in the United States: Initial Findings* (Denver: University of Colorado Center for Health Services Research, November 1985), p. I-12.

a. Excludes states that had no swing-bed hospitals during this period.

b. Provided medicaid reimbursement for swing-bed care at both the skilled and intermediate levels as of late 1984 or early 1985.

c. Based on July 1984 data due to temporary record-keeping problems at the Kansas HCFA Office.

d. Medicaid swing-bed reimbursement at the skilled level only.

by the hospital, exclusive of those for newborns, those in intensive-
care units, and those in nursing home distinct parts.

In what has proved to be a controversial decision, HCFA
interprets this provision to include hospitals licensed for more

than fifty beds if the hospital is staffed for only forty-nine or fewer beds. Thus some hospitals with more than fifty licensed beds may participate in the program. "Mothballed" beds are not counted. In order to participate in medicare and medicaid, the hospital must obtain a certificate of need for the provision of skilled nursing facility (SNF) or intermediate-care facility (ICF) services from the relevant state health planning and development agency.

Quality Standards

To ensure adequate quality of care, the Social Security Act requires that the SNF provisions governing discharge planning and social services apply to swing-bed hospitals. In addition, the statute requires that medicare SNF services in swing-bed hospitals "shall be subject to the same requirements applicable to such services when furnished by a skilled nursing facility except for those requirements the Secretary [of the Department of Health and Human Services] determines are inappropriate."[6] Implementing regulations require that in addition to meeting the standards of the Joint Commission on Accreditation of Hospitals or HCFA's conditions of participation, swing-bed hospitals must comply with the SNF conditions of participation for patients' rights, specialized rehabilitative services, dental services, social services, patient activities, and discharge planning.

Reimbursement

Medicare reimburses differently for routine care (that is, room, board, and nursing) and for ancillary services. Regardless of the actual costs incurred in furnishing routine SNF services in a participating swing-bed hospital, the statute specifies that routine services are to be reimbursed at the average medicaid SNF routine rate per day during the previous calendar year. Ancillary services (such as physical and occupational therapy) are reimbursed based on the proportion of total costs for the services accounted for by the medicare charges.

Reimbursement requirements for swing-bed long-term care days under medicare and medicaid were virtually identical until the Deficit Reduction Act of 1984 modified the medicaid provisions to allow states greater flexibility. States must, however, meet the general requirements of the Social Security Act, which stipulates that the method for reimbursement of skilled nursing and inter-

6. 42 U.S.C. 1395tt(f) (1985).

mediate-care facilities must be "reasonable and adequate to meet the costs which must be incurred by efficiently and economically operated facilities in order to provide care and services in conformity with applicable State and Federal laws, regulations, and quality and safety standards."[7] As a practical matter, however, most states follow the medicare reimbursement principles.

Conflicting Views

Since its inception, the swing-bed program has been very controversial. The hospital industry and other supporters of the program would like to see it expanded to include larger and more urban hospitals, especially those with low occupancy rates or a backlog of nursing home patients. In general, critics of the program, including nursing home groups, charge hospitals with using it to lessen the impact of medicare's DRG hospital prospective payment system. Some policymakers in the federal government worry that swing beds might represent double payment for services already covered in the DRG payment or that costs might rise out of control. Reflecting this controversy, conflicting bills on the subject have been introduced in Congress. One, by Representative Byron L. Dorgan, Democrat of North Dakota, would expand the swing-bed program to hospitals with fewer than 150 beds. Conversely, a bill by Representative Gerry Sikorski, Democrat of Minnesota, would impose significant new restrictions on the use of swing beds.

Issues addressed in this volume
In order to address the issues surrounding the use of swing beds, a conference was held at the Brookings Institution on February 24, 1986. The papers presented at this conference, which appear in revised form in this volume, examine a wide range of issues. My paper and the one by Kovner and Richardson lay out a framework for examining swing beds and summarize the experience of the Robert Wood Johnson Foundation demonstration. Turning first to economic and financial issues, Finkler analyzes the circumstances under which swing beds are cost effective, while Holahan examines several options for reimbursement reform. Turning next to the effect of swing beds on patients, Shaughnessy examines the effect of swing beds on access to nursing home care and Smits assesses the quality of care in swing beds. Finally, Vladeck presents the larger lessons of swing beds and implications for the future.

7. 42 U.S.C. 1396(a)(13)(A) (1985).

Overview of Policy Issues

I present an overview of policy issues concerning swing-bed hospitals raised by current law and the Robert Wood Johnson Foundation demonstration. I identify the major goals of the swing-bed program and several crosscutting themes that color the current policy debate. The major goals are improving patient access to nursing home services in rural areas, financially aiding rural hospitals, providing high-quality long-term care services, and providing services in a cost-effective setting and a cost-containing manner. These themes, generated by the different interests and perspectives of the nursing home industry, the hospital industry, government, and patients, are: (1) To what extent is it fair to exempt swing beds from certain requirements that nursing homes and distinct-part units of hospitals must meet? This theme is often put in terms of a conflict between maintaining a level playing field and maximizing program participation. (2) Should hospitals or freestanding nursing homes provide long-term care? (3) Do swing-bed patients receive a new service, or are they just renamed long-stay hospital patients? If the latter is true, does the swing-bed program result in double payment to hospitals for services already included in the medicare DRG payment? (4) Finally, in this time of budget austerity, does government really want to incur the cost of improved access to nursing home care?

Robert Wood Johnson Foundation Demonstration

Twenty-six swing-bed hospitals in five rural states were part of a national demonstration funded by the Robert Wood Johnson Foundation and administered through the Program in Health Policy and Management at New York University. As described in the paper by Kovner and Richardson, the Rural Hospital Program of Extended-Care Services began in April 1981 as an effort to promote the swing-bed concept by establishing models for small rural hospitals of how to provide high-quality, long-term care. As part of the demonstration, the hospitals received educational and technical assistance from their state hospital associations.

The program had four objectives. The first was to create an awareness and understanding of the opportunity afforded by the swing-bed provisions of medicare and medicaid reimbursement. A second objective was to show how the swing-bed concept can be implemented successfully by developing high-quality extended-care services to meet the special needs of chronically ill patients, instituting an internal quality assurance process, and strengthening financial management and third-party reimbursements. Third, by working with state hospital associations, the program sought to assist the development of technical assistance capabilities near the small rural hospitals. Finally, the program was designed so that the knowledge gained by the participants could be shared with others.

Based on the programwide data provided by the grantees, hospitals have been providing an increasing volume of short-term nursing home care at the skilled level of care. By the first quarter of 1985, demonstration hospital swing-bed patient-days represented 26 percent of total (acute and long-term care) patient-days. On average, each hospital had about twenty swing-bed admissions. The average length of stay was about twenty days. Almost three-fourths of the patients required skilled nursing. Medicare was the primary source of payment for 73 percent of all patients. Data on other swing-bed hospitals that are not part of the demonstration suggest roughly similar results. However, analyses by Shaughnessy and his colleagues suggest that these hospitals, on average, have fewer swing-bed patients and that fewer of their patients require skilled nursing and receive medicare benefits.[8]

Kovner and Richardson argue that the swing-bed program has resulted in the following benefits: (1) an increase in hospital staff sensitivity to the needs of the elderly; (2) an increase in availability of new services (such as physical therapy, social services, patient activities, and discharge planning) to all patients; (3) teaching staff new ways of working together; (4) a springboard for hospitals to diversify, particularly into other services for the elderly; (5) improved hospital finances through increased occupancy, higher revenues, better utilization of staff, more referrals, and improved physician recruitment; and (6) better care for patients by facilitating recovery near home, where the family can be closely involved with the patient's care.

Under What Conditions Are Swing Beds Cost Effective?

A key assumption in the rationale for swing beds is that the provision of long-term care in existing small rural hospitals is more cost effective than other alternatives for meeting the demand for nursing home care. In particular, the marginal cost of providing long-term care in low-occupancy rural hospitals is believed to be

8. Shaughnessy and others, *Hospital Swing Beds in the United States.*

less than in other settings because of the availability of surplus staff capacity and physical plant. In his paper, Steven Finkler attempts to test that hypothesis. He concludes that providing nursing home care in a new nursing home (including capital costs) would be 84 percent more expensive than in swing beds. In general, he suggests that incremental costs in hospitals are lower than total average costs in new nursing homes. Although a wide range of estimates are made, these conclusions would be reversed only if the estimates contained a significant and systematic bias in favor of the swing-bed alternative.

Finkler is careful to stress the limitations of his analysis. He notes that a key assumption is that there are no available nursing home beds. Therefore, the cost of providing long-term care in the hospital is compared with providing that care in a newly built nursing home bed. Finkler emphasizes that if there were excess capacity in existing nursing homes or if capacity could be increased in existing facilities, this would be the least expensive alternative. Moreover, by concentrating on a short-run analysis, he does not address the issue of the capital costs necessary when the swing-bed hospital needs replacement. In general, he disavows any assumption that all existing hospital beds should be replaced. In addition, ancillary costs, which prove to be substantial in swing-bed hospitals, are not included in the analysis.

Payment to Hospitals

Manipulation of medicare and medicaid reimbursement policy is one of the major levers decisionmakers have to achieve the goals of the swing-bed program. Under current law, medicare programs reimburse swing-bed skilled nursing facilities at the average state medicaid nursing home routine rate during the previous calendar year. Almost all medicaid programs also use this method to reimburse skilled nursing and intermediate care in swing-bed hospitals. In theory, this amount is supposed to cover the marginal cost of providing swing-bed services.

In his paper, John Holahan identifies reimbursement sufficient to encourage hospital participation in the swing-bed program as one of the principal objectives of the current swing-bed reimbursement system. Other objectives include encouraging access to high-quality care, minimizing administrative burdens for public programs and hospitals, paying facilities the same for serving similar patients regardless of the setting, and eliminating interstate differences in access to nursing home care.

In general, Holahan is negative about the current reimbursement system's ability to meet these objectives. Indeed, he argues that the current system meets few of these objectives other than administrative simplicity. It is unlikely to encourage participation in the swing-bed program over the longer term because it covers only variable and not total costs. Ironically, the use of existing hospital capital plant and staff, one of the principal rationales for swing beds, and the associated marginal cost pricing almost guarantee a relatively small program in terms of patients served and the swing-bed program's effect on access. Holahan argues that unless hospitals are reimbursed for their total average variable costs (including capital) over the long run, they will, at best, be able to afford to serve a very small number of patients and not even that during periods of peak acute-care occupancy. In addition, the system does not encourage access for heavy-care patients and provides no incentives for quality. Moreover, the dissimilarity in how nursing home patients are reimbursed in freestanding nursing homes, hospital-based skilled nursing facilities, and swing beds results in inequities across settings in payment for similar patients.

He analyzes a variety of possible reimbursement options, including continuing current policy, retrospective costs to a ceiling, retrospective costs to a case mix-adjusted ceiling, facility-specific rates with ceilings, prospective case mix-adjusted rates based on a facility case-mix index, and patient-specific case mix-adjusted rates. Choices among the options depend on how the policy priorities are weighed. Each option requires trade-offs among access, cost, and hospital participation.

Despite the deficiencies in the current system, it should be noted that current policy has provided somewhat improved access and has paid hospitals at a rate sufficient to entice more than half of eligible hospitals to participate. Indeed, based on Finkler's analysis, most hospitals appear to be reimbursed considerably above their marginal cost. Covering the full average costs of swing-bed care could vitiate the primary economic argument in favor of swing beds and might lead policymakers to prefer the construction of new nursing home beds instead.

Holahan acknowledges that his discussion does not address options for payment of ancillary services and the effect they would have on the policy objectives identified. In addition, although the focus on medicare is appropriate because it has been the major payer for swing-bed care, it should be recalled that private-pay patients account for a significant number of swing-bed patients.

Access

One of the major goals of the swing-bed program is to improve access to long-term care services by rural elderly. In his paper, Peter Shaughnessy, using data from the University of Colorado's ongoing evaluation of the national swing-bed program, concludes that access to institutional long-term care services for residents in rural communities has been increased by the availability of hospital swing beds.

Shaughnessy has three major findings. First, swing-bed hospitals have a somewhat higher proportion of patients with more intense medical and service needs than do freestanding nursing homes in comparable communities. Thus patients with more intense needs have better access to needed services. Second, swing beds appear to result in a net addition of services in rural areas, rather than a substitution of hospital-based nursing home services for freestanding ones. Third, a larger proportion of institutional long-term care patients received care in their home community after the presence of swing beds, and the distance traveled from home was less for swing-bed patients than for community nursing home patients. These facts suggest that elderly long-term care patients in rural communities are more likely to receive care in their home community if swing beds are available.

Shaughnessy's findings were limited only to the effect of swing beds on access to institutional long-term care and did not consider other community-based services such as home health care. Moreover, since the findings are not based on direct measures of access such as population-based utilization rates, the data presented can only be considered suggestive.

Quality of Care

Quality of care in swing-bed hospitals has proved to be a major issue. The evaluation of earlier demonstrations by Shaughnessy and associates found the quality of care in swing-bed hospitals to be somewhat lower than the quality of care provided in nursing homes.[9] Indeed, improving quality of care was a major focus of the Robert Wood Johnson demonstration. In her paper, Helen Smits identifies three components of quality in long-term care: basic medical and nursing services, functional assessment and rehabilitation efforts, and quality of life. The challenge to hospitals is to change their focus from the acute-care model of diagnosis-

---

9. Shaughnessy and others, *An Evaluation of Swing Bed Experiments*, vol. 1.

centered, largely physician-dominated care to the long-term care model, which is multidimensional and nurse centered.

Based on her site visits to several swing-bed hospitals and her participation on the demonstration advisory board, Smits suggests that it is easier for hospitals to do those aspects of long-term care most closely related to acute care, that is, meeting the basic medical and nursing needs of a medically intensive patient and providing services such as laboratory and diagnostic tests. She concludes that in areas outside of traditional acute-care roles, such as functional assessment and patient activities, swing-bed hospitals are deficient when compared with freestanding nursing homes. This is partially the result of the very small number of swing-bed patients served at any one time (usually only two or three), which makes it difficult for staff to "change gears" to organize adequate patient activities or otherwise meet the psychosocial needs of long-term care patients. Swing-bed hospitals also lack the critical mass of patients to carry out successful patient activities or to justify hiring some specialized staff.

The Meaning of Swing Beds

What has been learned from the swing-bed experience? In his paper, Bruce Vladeck argues that swing beds provide the basis for a thoroughgoing reassessment of the roles hospitals should play in the health care system in the future. Proclaiming swing beds to be a success, he is favorable to expanding them to urban areas and to other services like mental health. He suggests that there are three lessons and one fundamental principle that can be derived from swing beds.

The first lesson is that even relatively small and resource-poor hospitals can do, reasonably well, things they had not done before. In other words, hospitals can adapt to new demands. Second, the experience of swing beds demonstrates that sunk capital is cheaper than new, and fixed overhead costs can be spread more broadly than they generally are. In other words, services added at the margin may incur only marginal costs. With a hospital industry now operating well below optimal productive capacity, this may offer an opportunity to provide needed services at a somewhat lower cost than would otherwise be necessary. Third, the experience of swing beds indicates that it is desirable for people to receive services relatively close to home.

According to Vladeck, the fundamental principle is that institutions should fit the needs of the people they are supposed to serve, not the other way around. Institutional configurations should follow patient needs; real-life patients do not fit neatly into rigidly defined institutions. The very fact that the patient remains in the same institution over two or more levels of care is a consequential advantage in and of itself.

Not all, of course, accept his positive evaluation of the swing-bed experience. Commenting on Vladeck's paper, Stephen Press assesses the situation quite differently. He asserts that the essence of swing beds is "helping hospitals by sticking long-term care patients in their vacant beds." Moreover, he suggests that the cost arguments in favor of swing beds are bogus because hospitals fail to renovate their facilities to offer the social and recreational services that long-term care patients need. Services added at the margin may be insufficient to meet patient needs. Even worse, they may damage the communities' long-run interest by interfering with the development of a dependable community capacity to meet those needs. Swing beds, he argues, are a makeshift approach to long-term care.

Conclusion

In summary, the swing-bed concept has been reasonably successful in providing a needed service that was not previously available to the rural elderly in their own communities and that can benefit many small rural hospitals. The swing-bed concept is limited, however, in its potential to solve the problems of long-term care or rural hospitals. In particular, expanding the concept to much larger and more urban hospitals should be done cautiously. For these hospitals, demand for services and the availability of staff may be adequate for successful operation of full-fledged long-term care units that meet all of the usual requirements of hospital-based skilled nursing and intermediate-care facilities.

Swing beds seem to work best for patients who require short-stay, medically intensive services in small rural hospitals. It is not a program for all postacute patients or for all small rural hospitals. Nonetheless, by encouraging hospitals to use their excess capacity to meet community needs at a moderate cost, swing beds represent a useful approach to health policy.

Policy Issues

JOSHUA M. WIENER

IN EVALUATING any public policy, it is necessary to specify what a particular intervention is supposed to accomplish. Judgments about how well the swing-bed program is meeting its goals depend partially on whether swing beds are measured against acute-care hospitals without swing beds, new nursing homes, or existing nursing homes. In addition to asking whether goals are being met, one must look at the swing-bed program from the varying perspectives of different constituencies—the nursing home industry, the hospital industry, government, and patients and their families. There are several policy issues that are raised by these groups' needs and objectives.

Policy goals The swing-bed program has four major goals: improving patient access to nursing home services in rural areas; financially aiding rural hospitals; providing high-quality long-term care; and providing services in a cost-effective setting and in a cost-containing manner. Not surprisingly, these goals sometimes conflict. For example, it may not be possible to provide financial aid to rural hospitals while pursuing a policy of cost containment. These trade-offs are the grist of political conflict, and striking a balance among these competing goals is what policymaking is all about.

Improved Access to Nursing Home Services

The principal rationale for swing beds, improving patient access to nursing home services, is built on two basic assumptions. First, there is an unmet demand or need for nursing home services in many rural communities that is unlikely to be met through existing nursing homes or the construction of new facilities. Second, it is socially and medically preferable to treat long-term care patients in their home communities where family and friends can easily visit instead of transferring them to nursing homes in more distant communities.[1]

1. Peter W. Shaughnessy and others, *An Evaluation of Swing Bed Experiments to Provide Long-Term Care in Rural Hospitals,* vol. 1 (Denver: University of Colorado Center for Health Services Research, March 1980).

13

Financial Aid to Rural Hospitals

Almost all rural communities want to maintain their local hospital in order to ensure the continued availability of acute care and the employment and other economic benefits that hospitals provide. The maintenance of rural hospitals can no longer be assumed because many are in serious financial trouble, more now than when the original swing-bed legislation was enacted or when the Robert Wood Johnson Foundation demonstration was initiated. By 1995, 500 or more rural hospitals may have closed.[2]

This financial pressure has been caused by the new medicare prospective payment system, the national trend to declining hospital utilization, and the economic depression in the farm belt. Rural hospitals have been especially hard hit because they start from very low occupancy rates (generally less than 50 percent) and shorter stays. Moreover, health care utilization typically declines during economic downturns as people postpone care because they cannot afford to pay physicians or hospitals. In this environment, swing beds offer an additional source of revenue to help sustain rural hospitals.

High-Quality, Long-Term Care

A basic assumption of the swing-bed concept is that small rural hospitals are capable of providing high-quality or at least adequate care to long-term patients. The evaluation of the earlier swing-bed demonstration identified quality of care as a significant issue.[3] In general, the quality of care provided in swing-bed hospitals was found to be somewhat lower than that provided in the comparison nursing homes. If swing-bed care had been compared with how long-stay patients are treated in acute-care hospitals without swing beds, swing-bed care might have appeared in a more favorable light. Nonetheless, this finding led Congress to impose certain quality requirements that were not part of the earlier demonstration, and the Robert Wood Johnson Foundation also sought to make quality assurance a major focus of its efforts.

Cost Effectiveness and Cost Containment

In this age of deficit reduction, cost containment has a very high priority. The provision of long-term care in existing rural

2. Cynthia Wallace, "Rural System Corrals Profits with 'Back-to-Basics' Approach," *Modern Healthcare*, vol. 15 (December 6, 1985), pp. 70–80.
3. Shaughnessy and others, *An Evaluation of Swing Bed Experiments.*

hospitals is assumed to be more cost effective than other alternatives in meeting the demand for nursing home care. In particular, the marginal cost of providing long-term care in low-occupancy rural hospitals should be less than in other settings because of the availability of surplus staff and physical plant. Swing beds may appear cost effective against newly constructed nursing home beds, but not every nursing home bed in areas with swing-bed hospitals is completely full. The marginal cost of an additional patient in an existing nursing home may be less than the marginal cost of a swing-bed patient. Financial incentives for nursing homes to increase their occupancy rates might meet the access and cost-containment goals of swing beds at lower costs.

Crosscutting themes

Some policy concerns cut across these goals, generated by the different constituencies and perspectives of the nursing home industry, the hospital industry, government, and patients. It is a policy truism that "where you stand depends on where you sit."

A Level Playing Field versus Maximum Participation

The first major theme is whether it is fair to promote hospitals' participation in the swing-bed program by exempting them from some of the medicare and medicaid requirements that nursing homes must meet. This is a major point of contention for the nursing home industry, which maintains that such an exemption makes the playing field uneven.

Although they do have to meet all of the requirements of the Joint Commission on the Accreditation of Hospitals or HCFA's conditions of participation for hospitals, swing-bed hospitals do not have to meet the specific skilled nursing facility conditions of participation for state and local laws, governing body (except for patient rights), medical direction, physician services, nursing services, dietetic services, pharmaceutical services, physical environment, specialized rehabilitative services, outpatient physical therapy, laboratory and radiologic services, medical records, transfer agreements, infection control, disaster preparedness, and utilization review (except discharge planning). Similar but not identical requirements exist for general hospitals. The SNF requirement for separate dining and patient activity rooms is also not applied since this would require extensive structural modifications in many hospitals.

From the point of view of hospitals, easing these administrative and regulatory requirements is a necessary precondition to achieving program participation. From the point of view of nursing homes, it is unfair to make them meet requirements, fill out forms, and incur expenses that swing-bed hospitals do not.

When the implementing regulations were being written, the hospital industry strenuously argued that the only requirements that swing-bed hospitals should have to meet were the two specifically mentioned in the statute, discharge planning and social services. Given that during the swing-bed demonstration each hospital averaged only about two patients a day, they suggested that it would be "ludicrous" to require the full conditions of participation.

As a practical matter, swing-bed hospitals have a bit more regulatory flexibility in how they treat patients than do freestanding nursing homes. These exemptions from some of the conditions of participation are also a general recognition that the staffing problems of rural areas may make it difficult to apply the conditions of participation envisioned for more urban areas. Finally, as Helen Smits suggests in her paper, state and federal inspectors "are much less concerned about the neglect or abuse of patients in hospitals and therefore approach inspection of swing beds with a more positive attitude than is the case in many nursing homes."

From the perspective of the nursing home industry, this approach to the conditions of participation establishes a double standard: a higher one for nursing homes and a lower one for swing-bed hospitals. The exemption from some of the quality standards is particularly galling to the nursing home industry because it sends a subliminal message that hospitals can be "trusted" to provide adequate care without regulation, but nursing homes cannot. This seems especially unfair to them because of the demonstration evaluation findings referred to above. Moreover, if the urban model is inappropriate for swing-bed hospitals, then it is inappropriate for rural freestanding nursing homes as well.

Similarly, in terms of reimbursement, since medicare and most medicaid reimbursement for routine services is the average medicaid rate for the previous calendar year, hospitals have reduced accounting and cost-reporting burdens. This simplified approach has been justified primarily on the low number of swing-bed patients per hospital. On the other hand, in terms of medicare patients, the average swing-bed caseload is no less than the average caseload for 1,500 low-volume freestanding nursing homes that have to fill out the entire medicare SNF cost report.[4]

4. U.S. Department of Health and Human Services, Health Care Financing Administration, "Study of the Medicare Skilled Nursing Facility Benefit under Medicare," Report to Congress (HCFA, 1985).

Who Should Provide Long-Term Care?

The second major theme concerns the conditions under which swing beds are to be used. In its narrowest form, the question is whether swing beds should be used as full-fledged nursing homes or should be limited to holding patients only until they can be placed in freestanding nursing homes. More broadly, the issue is whether long-term care will remain predominantly in freestanding nursing homes or whether it will increasingly be provided by hospitals. As it has been debated, especially at state levels, the issue often appears to an outsider to be a fairly crude battle over market share.

In terms of providing care, hospitals assert that they provide the care that the freestanding nursing homes cannot or will not. Nursing homes are reluctant to participate in medicare because of low payment rates, retroactive denials, and burdensome reporting requirements.[5] As a result, medicare beneficiaries often find it difficult to gain access to skilled nursing facility services. In addition, hospital groups say SNFs are reluctant to take medicare patients because they have higher care needs and are more expensive to treat. The shortage of SNF beds is becoming even more severe because of the DRG incentives to discharge patients as early as possible.

From the hospital's perspective, swing beds can be used as an additional source of revenue to improve the financial condition of small, low-occupancy hospitals. According to Richardson and Kovner, "In the few hospitals where there has been an attempt to isolate the costs of swing-bed services, it has been found that the introduction of the swing-bed program did generate additional revenue that had an overall positive impact on hospital operations by reducing deficits or slightly increasing a surplus."[6] Indeed, Robert Wood Johnson Foundation demonstration hospitals are quite dependent on swing-bed patients, who account for approximately one-fifth of all patient-days provided by the hospitals. Shaughnessy and associates, however, are cautious in assessing how much of an effect swing beds can have on the financial viability of rural hospitals.[7] Noting that an average hospital had only two patients a day in swing-bed status, their evaluation of the earlier demonstration showed little discernible effect on the financial position of hospitals.

5. Ibid.
6. Hila Richardson and Anthony Kovner, "Implementing Swing-Bed Services in Small Rural Hospitals," *Journal of Rural Health*, vol. 2 (January 1986), pp. 52–53.
7. Shaughnessy and others, *An Evaluation of Swing Bed Experiments*, vol. 1.

From the nursing homes' perspective, however, some hospitals are inappropriately using swing beds to lessen the blow of medicare's new hospital prospective payment system.[8] The HCFA interpretation that allows hospitals with more than fifty licensed beds to participate in the swing-bed program especially raises concerns that hospitals will use swing beds even if nursing home beds are available in the community. Under the current system, hospitals can bypass making arrangements with nursing homes for discharged patients since they essentially operate their own SNF. The nursing home industry also has long been concerned with the quality of care in hospitals operating swing beds and charges that hospitals are not equipped or staffed to provide the kind of care and social interaction provided in community nursing homes. Nursing homes maintain that swing beds should be used as a temporary alternative for caring for a long-term care patient when community nursing home beds are not available, not as a financial rescue plan for hospitals that want to shift back and forth between acute care and long-term care depending on occupancy levels and financial need.

New Service or New Name?

While the previous two themes highlight conflicts between the hospital and nursing home industries, the third issue primarily affects government and the swing-bed hospitals. The advantage of swing beds is that hospitals can continue to treat patients after they are no longer in need of acute care without having to move them, in an often traumatic transfer, to a nursing home. This, however, raises the question of whether swing-bed patients receive a new service or whether their care is indistinguishable from that of long-stay acute-care patients awaiting placement in nursing homes.

Supporters of swing beds insist that swing-bed care is a "new" service. Although the conditions of participation that swing-bed hospitals must meet are not as specific as those for freestanding nursing homes, there is still a significant number of requirements, some of which (such as social work, patient activities, and dental care) require new staff or new contracting with outside personnel.

Indeed, a major argument in favor of expanding the program is that patients receive better care as swing-bed patients than they do as long-stay patients in a hospital where residents are treated

8. Stephanie Tames, "Hospitals, Nursing Homes Clash over Swing Beds," *Long Term Care Management,* vol. 14 (June 20, 1985), pp. 4–5.

as acute-care patients. While there is no systematic evidence available, there are anecdotal reports that care of long-stay patients is less than optimal (for example, nursing homes complain that some patients they admit from hospitals have bedsores because they have not been turned by hospital staff). Moreover, expansion of the swing-bed program might be a partial solution to the current DRG-created problem of hospitals being overly zealous in discharging patients (often called the "quicker and sicker" phenomenon). By receiving a modest additional payment, hospitals may be a little slower to discharge patients into less than optimal care arrangements.

Critics, on the other hand, are reminded of Senator George Aiken's solution to the Vietnam War. His approach was to declare victory and to withdraw from Vietnam as quickly as possible. By analogy, there is an acknowledged problem in acute-care hospitals of placing patients requiring nursing home care in rural (and urban) areas. The swing-bed solution is simply to declare back-logged patients "placed" in a swing bed without having to provide much in the way of new or different services. Thus, by renaming the patient, the problem is solved.

This issue is of more than just semantic interest because hospitals receive additional payment for swing-bed patients from the time that the hospital "discharges" the patient from the acute level of care to the long-term level of care. If the patient is merely an acute-care patient awaiting placement in a nursing home, additional payment does not begin until the "outlier" threshold is reached, a point fully three standard deviations beyond the geometric mean length of stay. Thus there is the potential for hospitals to "game" the system and maximize revenue by prematurely discharging patients into nursing home status.[9] While the peer review organizations are closely reviewing swing-bed admissions, the fact is that "premature discharge" is a nebulous concept, given the great variations in medical practice.

From the point of view of government, the issue is whether reimbursement for swing beds constitutes double payment. As an internal HCFA document noted:

> To expand the swing-bed program would be to aggravate further an existing "windfall" or "overpayment" problem which we have under the prospective payment system (PPS). The Federal portion and particularly the hospital specific portion of PPS rates include the costs

9. "Rural Hospitals Sanctioned for Abuse of Swing Bed Plan," *Modern Healthcare*, vol. 16 (January 3, 1986), p. 31.

of alternative placement days (APDs). Those APDs are days for which Medicare paid . . . because of the unavailability of SNF beds. In any case where a PPS hospital begins officially providing SNF care . . . subsequent to the base years used for computing the PPS rates, the hospitals will be able to get Medicare SNF payment for a substantial amount of care for which Medicare is already making "hospital" payment.[10]

In other words, a significant but unknown number of days of care at the nursing home level is already included in the DRG payment.

While swing beds may be a way for rural hospitals to increase their revenue by billing for an additional service not covered by the hospital prospective payment system, supporters of swing beds insist that this is no different than what is done for many other services. In particular, discharge to a freestanding nursing home or to a distinct-part nursing home unit in a hospital results in the same type of "double payment," yet few argue that the distinct-part or the freestanding nursing home should not be reimbursed. It is also financially indistinguishable from sending the patient home and providing home health services or seeing the patient after discharge in an outpatient department of a hospital. This type of activity is inevitable in a system where providers do not receive a fixed payment to cover all services. To the extent that hospitals move services to areas not covered by prospective payment, this fact should be reflected when the DRG payment rates are recalibrated.

Critics charge that consistent with the notion of double payment and gaming to maximize revenue is the very short long-term care that most swing-bed patients receive. Seventy percent of swing-bed patients in the Robert Wood Johnson Foundation demonstration had lengths of stay of less than twenty days, and 43 percent had lengths of stay of less than ten days.[11] In addition, 72 percent of patients in the demonstration had their care paid for by medicare. By comparison, only about 2 percent of total nursing home revenues come from medicare.[12] These results are roughly consistent with findings from the earlier HCFA demonstrations.[13]

---

10. Memorandum, Henry R. Desmarais to Patrice Hirsch Feinstein, "Subject: Discussion Paper: Extension of Swing-Bed Option," HCFA, May 23, 1984.

11. Data from quarterly reports of grantee hospitals to the Robert Wood Johnson Demonstration Program.

12. Katharine R. Levit and others, "National Health Expenditures, 1984," *Health Care Financing Review*, vol. 7 (Fall 1985), pp. 1–35.

13. Shaughnessy and others, *An Evaluation of Swing Bed Experiments*, vols. 1, 2.

Thus swing beds are rarely used for patients with extremely long lengths of stay.

Beyond the gaming issue, medicare program administrators are clearly worried that a large portion of medicare hospital patients may go through a period where they could reasonably qualify for medicare SNF benefits but are not likely to be so categorized unless the hospital has a financial incentive to so classify them. Thus expansion of the swing-bed program to larger and more urban hospitals could have significant fiscal implications for medicare.

Does Government Really Want to Improve Access to Nursing Home Care?

The fourth theme reflects the conflict between government and patients. The heavy financial involvement of medicare and medicaid in long-term care, coupled with the large potential demand for care in the community, means that increases in the nursing home supply translate directly into increased public expenditures. Thus there is a tension between cost containment and improved access to care.

While the current expenditures for the swing-bed program are small, expansion of the concept to larger and more urban hospitals raises the possibility of more substantial expenditures. On the one hand, results from the earlier swing-bed demonstration seem to suggest that there is a real need for more nursing home services, especially medicare-funded skilled nursing care. In a study of South Dakota, Shaughnessy and Tynan note, "The empirical results indicate that the long term care utilization experience of swing-bed hospitals was not caused by the diversion of long-term care patients from existing nursing homes, but instead represented a demand that previously had not been met."[14] Medicare-funded skilled nursing facility beds account for only 14 percent of nursing home beds in states with twenty-three or more swing-bed hospitals, compared with 31 percent in the country as a whole.[15] Thus it appears that many rural communities may be in need of additional long-term care beds.

On the other hand, fiscal pressures have led governments to impose a variety of mechanisms to try to constrain the nursing home supply. The federal government faces $200 billion deficits

14. Peter W. Shaughnessy and Eileen A. Tynan, "The Use of Swing Beds in Rural Hospitals," *Inquiry*, vol. 22 (Fall 1985), p. 313.

15. HCFA, "Health Facilities Participating in Health Care Financing Administration Programs, 1985," *Health Care Financing Review*, vol. 6 (Summer 1985), pp. 143–47.

and the deus ex machina of Gramm-Rudman-Hollings. State governments will soon feel the effects of those budget cuts unless Congress and the president can come to some agreement about alternative strategies for deficit reduction. In addition, twelve states had moratoriums on new nursing home beds in 1985 as a way of trying to control their medicaid expenditures.[16] Controlling the supply is a major avenue of controlling costs, at least in the short term.

Finally, although there is a perception of shortages of nursing home care in rural areas, it should be noted that the rural states have some of the highest ratios of nursing home beds to population in the country. For example, compared with a national average of 57.5 beds per 1,000 people age 65 and over in 1980, predominantly rural South Dakota had 94.2 beds per 1,000 elderly, Iowa had 86.4, Kansas had 81.5, and Colorado had 69.4.[17] These are among the highest nursing home bed ratios in the country. There may be other areas in the country with a more pronounced shortage of nursing home beds.

Conclusion

The swing-bed program generates policy conflict on at least three different levels. First, there is a relatively narrow debate over how well swing beds meet their policy goals of improving the lot of rural elderly and hospitals. The quality of care provided in swing beds is probably the most important area of concern. Second, there is a somewhat broader debate among hospitals, nursing homes, and government that is cast in terms of equity among providers, market share, and financial responsibility. This debate cuts across some of the narrower goals.

What is interesting about swing beds, however, is that the intensity of the debate far exceeds what would be expected, given the very small amount of reimbursement and number of patients actually involved. Debate over swing beds is often quite passionate. This intensity exists because swing beds raise fundamental questions about how the acute- and long-term care systems should be organized and financed. Should institutions provide a continuum of care, or should they specialize? What is the appropriate setting for the provision of long-term care? What should be the role of hospitals in health care? How should hospitals respond to the medicare prospective payment system and other cost containment

16. Intergovernmental Health Policy Project, George Washington University, personal communication, September 1985.

17. U.S. National Center for Health Statistics, *Health, United States, 1984* (Government Printing Office, December 1984), p. 134.

initiatives? Can and should rural hospitals be saved from financial collapse? All of these questions are likely to become more common as the health care system increasingly must cope with the chronic disabilities of the elderly and the unrelenting cost containment initiatives of government and other third-party payers.

The Robert Wood Johnson Demonstration Program

ANTHONY R. KOVNER
and HILA RICHARDSON

IN THE EARLY 1970s many rural areas lacked sufficient extended-care services, particularly those provided by skilled nursing homes, to meet local care needs. Local nursing homes were often characterized by high occupancy rates and waiting lists for admissions.[1] Families became separated when patients had to be admitted to nursing homes many miles from their homes.

The origins of this situation, in part, lay in the reimbursement requirements of the federal medicare and medicaid programs. Many small rural hospitals once provided acute and long-term care in the same facility. When medicare and medicaid were introduced, however, they required that hospitals be certified to provide long-term care, and this care had to be provided in a physically distinct part of the institution used exclusively for that purpose. In addition, these separate areas had to include facilities for such specialized services as physical therapy, social services, and activities programs that assist patients to become or remain ambulatory. These policies prompted many hospitals to stop providing long-term care.

At the same time, the occupancy rates for many rural hospitals were declining because of a shrinking population base, inadequate physician supply, and loss of patients to referral centers in urban areas.[2] This decline in rural hospital occupancy, combined with the shortage of extended-care beds in rural areas, led the federal government to sponsor an experimental program to determine whether hospital swing beds could offer a satisfactory response. From 1973 to 1981, a total of 108 rural hospitals in Iowa, South Dakota, Texas, and Utah participated in this federal demonstra-

---

1. Based on data from the U.S. Social Security Administration, Office of Research and Statistics, 1974.

2. Based on American Hospital Association data, 1980. Also see Roger A. Rosenblatt and Ira S. Moscovice, *Rural Health Care* (Wiley, 1982).

tion, which was evaluated by the University of Colorado Center for Health Services Research.[3]

The evaluators described problems encountered by demonstration hospitals as largely centering around issues of reimbursement and orientation of hospital staff, which could have been avoided or overcome if the participating hospitals had shared information more widely and had been provided with adequate technical assistance. Nonetheless, the evaluators recommended the implementation of a national swing-bed program based on these major findings:

—An unmet need for extended-care services existed in many rural communities.

—The provision of long-term care in existing rural hospitals was potentially more cost effective than other alternatives in meeting the demand for extended-care services.

—Patients and families benefited when patients stayed in their communities for nursing home care.

—Rural hospitals could improve their financial condition by providing swing-bed services.

Primarily because of this experimental effort, Congress enacted provisions in the Omnibus Reconciliation Act of 1980 allowing medicare and medicaid payment for swing-bed care in rural hospitals if they had fewer than fifty beds, had received a certificate of need (if required by the state), and had made provisions to provide social services, patient activities, discharge planning, and special rehabilitation services to their long-term care patients. The hospitals are paid at the average rate per day that the given state's medicaid plan paid last year to nursing homes for routine services. Ancillary services are billed separately on a cost basis.

Congress, however, did not provide support for hospitals to obtain education and technical assistance for meeting the special nursing care and administrative requirements that can be barriers to implementation of a swing-bed program. The Rural Hospital Program of Extended-Care Services (Swing-Bed) of the Robert Wood Johnson Foundation (RWJ), cosponsored by the American Hospital Association, was planned to meet this need. It is a five-year demonstration program that has granted more than $6 million to help hospital associations and hospitals implement the swing-bed concept.

3. Peter W. Shaughnessy and others, *An Evaluation of Swing Bed Experiments to Provide Long-Term Care in Rural Hospitals*, vol. 2 (Denver: University of Colorado Center for Health Services Research, March 1980).

The RWJ demonstration

The Rural Hospital Program of Extended-Care Services has been conducted in two phases: in the first phase, which lasted from January 1982 to December 1985, five state hospital associations each received grants of up to $300,000 over four years to offer technical assistance to rural hospitals interested in developing swing-bed operations. In the second phase, from January 1983 to December 1986, twenty-six rural hospitals in the five states each received grants of up to $200,000 over four years to implement the swing-bed concept. In addition to support for the state hospital associations and the hospitals, RWJ gave a grant to the American Hospital Association, the program's cosponsor, to develop a national communications and education effort.

The program has been administered through the Program in Health Management and Policy at New York University under the direction of Anthony R. Kovner. A program advisory committee assisted in the reviews of applications and in monitoring the progress of the program. It is currently being evaluated by the University of Colorado Center for Health Services Research under the direction of Peter W. Shaughnessy.

Objectives

The program has four objectives. The first is to create an awareness and understanding of the opportunity afforded by the swing-bed provisions of medicare and medicaid reimbursement. A second objective is to show how small rural hospitals can implement the swing-bed concept successfully by developing high-quality extended-care services to meet the special needs of chronically ill patients; instituting an internal quality assurance process; and strengthening financial management and third-party reimbursements. Third, by working with state hospital associations, the program seeks to assist in developing capabilities for technical assistance near the small rural hospitals. And finally, the program was designed so that the knowledge gained by its participants can be shared with others to further implement the swing-bed concept nationally.

Grantees

Funding was made available on a competitive basis to five of the twenty-four eligible state hospital associations: Kansas, Missouri, New Mexico, North Dakota, and Mississippi. Hospital associations were eligible if they were in states that: (1) had 35 percent or more of their population in nonmetropolitan areas; (2) had at least ten acute-care hospitals in nonmetropolitan areas; and

Table 1. *Characteristics of Grantee Hospitals, 1981*

Characteristic	Number (n = 26)	Characteristic	Number (n = 26)
Number of beds		*Management*	
Less than 20	2	Community	14
20–29	5	Hospital system	4
30–40	6	Church-operated	6
41–50	9	Larger hospital	2
More than 50	4	Hospitals with distinct parts	4
Occupancy rates (percent)		*Payer (percent)*[a]	
25–40	7	Medicare	
41–54	14	Less than 20	2
55–75	5	20–50	12
Ownership		51 or more	11
Community	8	Medicaid	
County or city	11	Less than 10	19
Hospital district	2	11–29	6
Church-owned	4	Blue Cross or commercial	
Hospital-owned	1	insurance	
		Less than 20	3
		21–50	20
		51 or more	2

Source: Data from quarterly reports of grantee hospitals to the Robert Wood Johnson Demonstration Program.
a. Payer information was not available on one of the grantee hospitals.

(3) had not participated in the earlier federal demonstration. The associations were to offer technical assistance to eligible hospitals in their state in three areas: marketing and the establishment of eligibility; professional services to help hospital staff learn how to meet the special needs of the chronically ill patients and their families; and financial management.

Of the twenty-six hospitals that received funding, six were in Kansas, six in New Mexico, five in Missouri, five in North Dakota, and four in Mississippi. A summary of their characteristics when they entered the program is provided in table 1. To be eligible for a grant, a hospital had to: (1) be located in one of the five grantee states; (2) have fewer than fifty acute-care beds; (3) be a short-term not-for-profit or state or locally owned general hospital; (4) be located in a nonmetropolitan area; (5) make a commitment of at least five acute-care beds or swing beds (this was later changed to 10 percent of acute beds); (6) make a formal commitment to serve patients without regard to race, sex, or economic circumstances; and (7) designate a professional staff member with appropriate qualifications to be responsible for implementing the swing-bed project.

In order for hospitals to demonstrate a formal commitment to the program, the hospital's trustees had to agree to participate in the program and to continue swing-bed services after expiration of the foundation's grant, and the medical staff had to agree to the hospital's participation in the program and to its proposed swing-bed services. By the time the grant was made and before payment could begin, the hospital had to meet medicare and medicaid conditions of participation.

Once certified, the hospitals could use grant funds for training and salary assistance to replace staff being trained, salary assistance for staff to provide specialized services such as physical therapy, recruitment of volunteers, implementing a system for quality assurance, public education, and physical therapy and rehabilitation equipment (up to $10,000). Grant funds could not be used to replace existing budgets for services to the chronically ill, reimbursement of direct patient services, or the construction or renovation of facilities.

Data from the demonstration hospitals

The following discussion is based on the quarterly reports from the grantee hospitals from January 1983 through June 1985. In addition to patient data, the reports contain information on reimbursement, quality assurance, special services, and problems related to swing-bed service.

Swing-Bed Utilization

Hospital swing-bed patient-days increased steadily during the first two and one-half years of the demonstration, while acute-care patient-days declined.[4] During the first quarter of 1983, when the hospitals were beginning the program, there were 1,526 swing-bed patient-days in all grantee hospitals, or an average of 59 patient-days per hospital. One year later, swing-bed patient-days had increased to 8,522 for all grantee hospitals, for an average of 327 patient-days. Between the first quarters of 1984 and 1985, the increase in swing-bed patients was less than in the previous year, but the total swing-bed patient-days rose to 10,221, an average of close to 400 per hospital.

During the same period the grantee hospitals experienced a 20 percent decline in acute-care patient-days. The influence of swing-bed patient-days on total patient-days, therefore, has become increasingly important during the grant. In the first quarter of 1983, for example, swing-bed patient-days were 3 percent of total

4. The data from the demonstration hospitals presented in this section are from quarterly data submitted by each hospital from January 1983 through June 1985. The hospitals have reported on admissions, discharges, sociodemographic characteristics, and functional status of patients receiving swing-bed services on the last day of the quarter.

patient-days. In the first quarter of 1984, swing-bed patient-days had become 19 percent of the total, and by the first quarter of 1985, they had grown to 26 percent.

The stabilizing effect that swing-bed days have had on grantee hospital occupancy is further illustrated by a comparison of occupancy rates of the grantees in the five states in 1981, before swing-bed services were implemented, with occupancy rates in 1984 and the first half of 1985, with and without swing-bed days. Between 1981 and 1984, the acute-care occupancy rate dropped in the grantee hospitals in every state, from a 50 percent decrease in Kansas to a 25 percent decrease in Missouri. However, when swing-bed days are counted, the decline in the occupancy rate of Kansas grantee hospitals is reduced to only 21 percent and in Missouri to only 13 percent. In two states, Mississippi and North Dakota, swing-bed patient-days increased the total occupancy rate of the grantee hospitals in 1984 to a rate higher than in 1981, before swing-bed services began.

The same trend in occupancy has continued between 1984 and the first two quarters of 1985. Total occupancy in grantee hospitals has declined, with total acute-care occupancy falling below 35 percent. Counting swing-bed patient-days increases the total occupancy by 7 to 17 percent, raising total occupancy to 35–40 percent in three states and above 45 percent in the other two.

The average length of stay for skilled-care and intermediate-care swing-bed patients in the grantee hospitals has remained fairly constant, with a low of 15.6 days in the first quarter of 1983 and a high of 25.2 days in the third quarter of 1983. At the end of the 1984 grant year, the average length was 21.2 days, and it fell slightly to 19.8 days during the first quarter of 1985.

Since average length of stay has remained relatively stable, the increase in swing-bed patient-days is largely accounted for by the steady growth in swing-bed admissions. In the first quarter of 1983, there was a total of 98 patients in all the hospitals, or an average of 4 patients per grantee hospital, admitted for swing-bed services. In the first quarter of 1984, the total of swing-bed patients admitted had quadrupled to 394 patients, or an average of 15 in each hospital, and by the first quarter of 1985 there were 522 total admissions, or an average of 20.

Swing-Bed Patient Characteristics

The characteristics of the typical swing-bed patient have remained relatively unchanged over the duration of the program (see table 2). The typical patient is a white, female widow who

Table 2. *Selected Characteristics of Swing-Bed Patients in Grantee Hospitals, June 30, 1985*

Characteristic	Percent (n = 501)ᵃ	Characteristic	Percent (n = 501)ᵃ
Age		*Location before admission*	
Under 65	6.6	Private residence	
65–74	24.6	Alone	28.3
75–84	38.9	With family	52.1
Over 85	29.9	Acute-care hospital	8.0
Race		Other facility	11.6
White	89.1	*Primary reason for admission*	
Black	7.2	Fracture	13.6
Hispanic	2.6	Stroke	12.2
American Indian	1.2	Neoplasms	11.8
Sex		Disease of respiratory system	11.0
Female	57.5	Heart disease	9.6
Male	42.5	Other	41.8
Level of care		*Status after discharge*	
Skilled	74.8	Private residence	
Intermediate	24.3	Alone	11.5
Other extended care	0.8	With family	38.6
Source of payment		Skilled nursing facility	11.3
Medicare	60.7	Intermediate-care facility	11.7
Medicaid	6.8	Acute-care hospital	11.3
Medicare/medicaid	12.9	Other institution	1.5
Self-pay	16.9	Death	10.5
Other	2.8	Other	3.6

Source: See table 1.

a. Due to reporting problems, the total number of patients varies slightly among categories. The percentages are based on the number of patients reporting in each category and may not add to 100 due to rounding.

is 75 years or older and requires a skilled-nursing level of care, which is covered by medicare. The patient is initially admitted to the hospital from a private residence where she has been living alone or with family members. The most common reason for admission to acute care is a fracture or a stroke. During their swing-bed stay, about half the patients receive physical therapy. Upon discharge, there is slightly more than a 50 percent chance that the swing-bed patient will return to live alone or with family members and a 23 percent chance that the patient will be discharged to a nursing home. Readmission to an acute level of care occurs about 11 percent of the time, and about 10 percent of the patients die while at a swing-bed level of care.

Reimbursement for Swing-Bed Services

The hospitals in the demonstration have been paid for routine swing-bed services, as stipulated in the authorizing legislation, using a per diem rate based on the average state medicaid skilled or intermediate care rate for the previous year plus the reasonable cost of ancillary services. The average skilled and intermediate rates in 1985 for the five states ranged from a low of $35.87 to a high of $69.71 for skilled care and a low of $28.62 to a high of $43.03 for intermediate-level care. Grantee hospitals report that ancillary charges average between $30 to $50 per swing-bed patient-day.

At the end of the second quarter of 1985, 61 percent of the swing-bed patients were covered under medicare, 17 percent were self-paying, 13 percent were medicare with medicaid paying coinsurance, and 7 percent were covered under the state's medicaid plan. The remaining 3 percent of the swing-bed patients were covered by other insurance or pension plans. The combined medicare and medicare-medicaid swing-bed patients accounted for 74 percent of all patients, making the swing-bed program in the grantee hospitals largely a medicare program. Most of the patients in the self-paying category no longer require medicare skilled-nursing care and do not meet the state's criteria for medicaid eligibility to cover their stay at an intermediate level of care.

The financial effect of swing beds on the hospitals has not been fully documented largely because the cost-accounting methods used in the hospitals cannot adequately identify the incremental cost associated with swing-bed patient care. In the few hospitals where there has been an attempt to isolate the costs of swing-bed services, the introduction of the swing-bed program did bring in additional revenue that had an overall positive effect on hospital operations by reducing deficits or slightly increasing a surplus. For example, using data from the first quarter of 1985, the average grantee hospital would have 1,570 swing-bed and 4,500 acute-care patient-days for a total of 6,000 patient-days in 1985. The revenue for each swing-bed patient-day was, on average, $87: $47 for routine services and $40 for ancillary charges. This would provide a total of $136,590 in annual swing-bed revenue. Assuming total hospital revenue is $2.25 million, at $375 per day for 6,000 days, swing-bed revenue is roughly 6 percent of total revenue. The revenue estimates vary depending on the volume and patient mix of both acute-care and swing-bed patients.

After October 1983 the grantee hospitals, like all U.S. hospitals, were phased in under the medicare prospective payment system for their acute-care patients. The new reimbursement method pays hospitals a certain amount, prospectively, depending on the diagnostic-related group (DRG) in which the patient fits. The hospital is paid the same amount no matter how long the patient remains in the hospital. Although DRGs are not used in paying for swing-bed services, the availability of swing-bed services under this reimbursement method has provided an indirect financial benefit to hospitals. With swing beds, when the patient requires long-term care the change can occur with only a paper transfer, instead of waiting for an available nursing home bed. Thus swing beds can be especially helpful to small rural hospitals in areas with shortages of skilled nursing beds.

Although the prospective payment system does create an incentive to discharge patients as soon as medically appropriate, each swing-bed admission is reviewed for appropriateness by the state professional review organization (PRO) *before* the hospital is reimbursed for services it has already provided. Therefore hospitals are discouraged from premature transfer of patients to swing beds because they risk having medicare or medicaid payment denied.

Summary of Data

Based on the programwide data provided by the grantee hospitals, the hospitals have been providing an increasing volume of relatively short long-term care to elderly patients who need a skilled level of care and receive a full range of rehabilitative services. The patients leave the hospitals within thirty days of admission to swing-bed care and usually return home to live alone or with their family. Payment for swing-bed services has been mainly through the medicare program and has provided a new source of revenue for the grantee hospitals. The effects of the revenue have not been fully determined and probably vary depending on the volume of patients, patient mix, and local hospital conditions.

The five case studies below will provide an in-depth look at how the swing-bed program has actually worked. The examples were selected to present a closer view of the benefits of the program at the state and hospital level. The cases are not intended to be comprehensive or typical of demonstration hospitals and hospital associations, but rather to show key aspects of the potential of the program.[5] The swing-bed program has not had the same effect in each grantee hospital association or hospital.

---

5. The authors have presented a more comprehensive review of the demonstration and its implementation problems in "Implementing Swing-Bed Services in Small Rural Hospitals," *Journal of Rural Health*, vol. 2 (January 1986), pp. 46–60.

The hospital association as provider of technical assistance

The Kansas Hospital Association was awarded a grant in February 1982. Of the state's 149 acute-care hospitals, 85, or almost 60 percent, have fewer than fifty beds. This is a greater number of eligible hospitals than in the other grantee states. Since only 6 of these 85 hospitals were grantees, Kansas is a good state to observe for the potential acceptance and widespread implementation of the swing-bed concept through technical assistance provided by the hospital association to hospitals not receiving special financial grant assistance.[6]

As expected, during the first three and one-half years of the program, the swing-bed concept grew very rapidly in Kansas. As of July 1985, of the hospitals with fewer than fifty beds, fifty-one, or 60 percent, were medicare-certified to provide swing-bed services. In addition, seventeen of the thirty-two hospitals with fifty to one hundred beds had been certified for swing-bed services.[7] These sixty-two hospitals (excluding the six grantees) have implemented swing-bed services without any special financial assistance. A recent telephone survey of one-third of the Kansas swing-bed hospitals not funded by RWJ revealed several ways in which the state hospital association has helped them start swing-bed programs.

—*Assistance with meeting conditions of participation*: The hospital association helped all eligible hospitals in Kansas to expedite the medicare certification process through early coordination with the Kansas Department of Health and Environment to obtain certificates of need and by assistance with development of protocols required before the review by survey and licensure personnel. The certification process has not been a barrier to eligible swing-bed hospitals in Kansas. Most hospitals were approved on the first survey visit. The few that were not approved initially had minor problems that were quickly corrected.

—*Assistance with reimbursement*: Once the swing-bed regulations were published, the hospital association moved quickly to get clarification on the billing and payment of swing-bed services. The association organized a training session for all hospitals on billing medicare and medicaid claims for swing-bed patients and

6. The information in the Kansas case study is based on a survey of swing-bed hospitals and interviews with state officials conducted by Jane Ford, swing-bed director at the Kansas Hospital Association.

7. The Health Care Financing Administration considers hospitals with more than forty-nine beds to be eligible for certification if a hospital can furnish documentation that it is using fewer than fifty beds. Failure to adhere to the agreement to use fewer than fifty beds could result in termination of the HCFA swing-bed approval for reimbursement.

wrote and distributed a pamphlet describing swing-bed reimbursement. The project director also conducted seminars to help hospitals understand the documentation necessary for approval of a skilled or intermediate swing-bed stay and provided on-site assistance to nursing staffs in hospitals with documentation problems. The director has helped the hospitals prepare for their first PRO review and assisted them with correcting any problems identified. The PRO reports that Kansas has a minimal denial rate for swing-bed days.

—*Assistance with implementation problems*: One of the main implementation problems that hospital administrators report is gaining the nursing staff's support for the swing-bed program. Nursing staffs have often resisted the additional and different responsibilities in the swing-bed program. They must learn to care for the chronically ill patient (a role an acute-care nurse may find frustrating and less interesting), become familiar with state and federal criteria for assessing levels of care, and learn to work with new specialists and become more involved with the patient's family. The hospital association has played a key role in addressing and minimizing staff resistance. Early in the program, the association contracted with a nurse educator and specialist in gerontological nursing who developed special educational programs to help nurses deal with their new responsibilities.

—*Working with the nursing home industry*: Within the first few months of the grant, the project director met with the executive directors of both the voluntary and for-profit nursing home associations in the state to explain the swing-bed program and discuss potential problems. Problems that have occurred have been mainly local and usually have stemmed from concern that the hospital will try to replace the nursing home and not return patients after hospitalization. However, local nursing home administrators are realizing the swing-bed program allows them to keep heavy-care patients until they are stabilized at an intermediate level of care. The nursing home administrators are also realizing that the swing-bed program indirectly benefits them by helping keep the hospital viable. If the local hospital closes, the nursing home not only loses an essential referral source, but also some or all of the physicians may leave the community and the nursing home itself may be threatened. On the state level, there was an unsuccessful attempt by the for-profit nursing home industry to require swing-bed hospitals to meet all the nursing home certification requirements. The concern of the for-profit nursing home industry about competition from swing-bed hospitals is not unfounded and will probably continue.

—*Promotional activities by the state hospital association*: Hospital administrators reported that among the reasons they started swing-bed services was the information they received from the Kansas Hospital Association about the benefits to the hospital and the community. The most common benefit they mentioned was being able to discharge patients to their homes after a recuperative period in a swing bed rather than keeping them at the acute-care level waiting for nursing home placement.

Effect on hospital services

The demonstration program has assisted small rural hospitals to change the way they provide acute care and to introduce new services to the hospital's acute-care patients, as well as to its short-stay long-term care patients. The experience of Cedar County Memorial Hospital, a thirty-four-bed facility in El Dorado Springs, Missouri, is representative of that of many of the twenty-six grantees in the RWJ demonstration program.[8]

Staff Sensitivity to Elderly Patients

The in-service educational programs provided as orientation to nursing and other staff at Cedar County Memorial Hospital have emphasized the psychosocial needs of the elderly. As a result, the nursing staff has changed some of the ways of caring for elderly patients, whether acute or long term. For example, instead of doing everything for patients, as is frequently the approach for short-term acute stays, the staff now takes the additional time necessary to allow many acute-care patients to dress and feed themselves. Also, the staff is more willing to vary from the hospital routine and let elderly patients maintain their usual routine. Another change has been to involve families with the patients' care. Family members are encouraged to come at meal and bath time to help the patient and can stay after visiting hours to help get the patient ready for sleep. This not only saves the nursing staff time, it also teaches the family members proper techniques for helping the immobile patient and makes the transition to home easier for the family of a patient who has special problems.

Availability of New Services to All Patients

For most small rural hospitals, the development of swing-bed services means the introduction of special services required by the conditions of participation: physical therapy, social services, pa-

8. The information in the case study of Cedar County Memorial Hospital was provided by Arlene Moomaw, administrator, and her staff, in particular Debbie Johnson, swing-bed project coordinator.

tient activities, and discharge planning. Cedar County had a physical therapist and social worker when the swing-bed program began. With swing-bed funding this hospital was able to add speech and occupational therapists. However, none of these services was used extensively for acute-care patients until the physicians had experience with them in the swing-bed program. Now physicians routinely refer acute-care patients to the social worker for discharge planning and use rehabilitative services for all patients at a greater rate. In addition, the nursing staff now evaluates the physical and mental functioning of all patients, using the assessment tools developed for the swing-bed patients. The hospital staff has also begun to appreciate the benefits of including the acute-care patients who need socialization or sensory stimulation in parties and other events planned for swing-bed patients.

New Ways of Staff Working Together

Swing-bed care requires that nurses and specialized staff take more responsibility for patient care, and the physician becomes less involved in the daily monitoring of the patients. Physicians, for example, do not always visit the long-term care patients daily and must rely on the assessment and observations of the nursing staff in detecting changes in the patients' status. Also, the nurse swing-bed coordinator or social service director makes the assessment or referrals for swing-bed services and makes care recommendations for long-term care patients to the physician, rather than vice versa. The physicians and nurses depend on the physical therapist's evaluation of patients' functional level and progress. The social worker must rely on observations from all disciplines in planning for timely and appropriate discharge. The increased communication and cooperation, which is necessary for all staff to fulfill their professional responsibility for the patient, has engendered a new mutual professional respect among the staff.

Provision of Other Services to the Elderly

The swing-bed program has also been a springboard for hospitals to diversify, particularly into other services for the elderly. The swing-bed program is often the first experience hospital staff and boards of trustees have with nontraditional hospital acute care. A successful experience with swing beds can make staffs and boards more receptive to trying new services. The swing-bed program also provides a core of specialized personnel, such as physical therapists and social workers, as resources to the hospital, which allows the hospital to offer a range of other services that can help compensate for the decrease in acute-care revenue. All grantee hospitals have received funding through the RWJ program to implement diversification projects targeted at the elderly. Cedar County is using the funds to develop a cardiac rehabilitation program. Other hospitals are developing home health, emergency response systems, meals-on-wheels, and screening and wellness programs.

Effect on hospital finances

District II, a twenty-nine-bed hospital in Durant, Mississippi, provides an example of the direct and indirect ways that the swing-bed program can help a hospital through a period of financial and organizational crisis.[9] District II is not typical of RWJ grantees: swing beds have played a much more significant part in its financial survival than in other grantee hospitals, where swing-bed revenues typically compose 5–10 percent of total hospital revenues.

In January 1983, when the grant was awarded to District II hospital, it was a twenty-nine-bed acute-care hospital with an average daily census of thirteen patients. One year later, in January 1984, the hospital had gone from a surplus of $34,000 to a deficit of $600,000, due to poor fiscal management by a new administrator. It had fifty-four employees, one of the highest numbers the hospital had ever had, but there were vacancies in nursing and ancillary personnel and overstaffing in nonpatient care areas such as the business office. The only on-site ancillary service was respiratory therapy. General lab, X-ray, and pharmacy services were provided by outside contractors. Physical therapy and social work were not available in the community. The hospital's average daily census had dropped from 13.5 to 8.7 patients due to substantial renovations and the resignation of two physicians.

With the implementation of the swing-bed program, the hospital's financial status improved substantially, even though the average number of acute-care patients did not change. Although other managerial and organizational changes also made a contribution, the swing-bed program had the following effects:

—*Increased hospital occupancy:* Since 1984 swing-bed patient-days have ranged from 38–40 percent of total patient-days at District II.

—*Increased revenue:* During the two and one-half years of the swing-bed program, the hospital generated approximately $252,000 in revenue from the swing-bed patients.

9. The information for the case study of District II Community Hospital was provided by Joe McLellan, administrator.

—*Better utilization of staff:* In July 1985, when there were two acute-care patients, the thirteen swing-bed patients increased the staffing needs by four to six people a day, allowing District II to avoid the additional lay-offs that many small rural hospitals have had to enforce.

—*Increased referrals:* With the availability of swing beds and physical therapy, both inpatient and outpatient, the hospital has become a referral center for swing-bed and rehabilitation patients from larger hospitals in Jackson, less than an hour away.

—*Improved physician perception of the hospital:* The program offers an additional and convenient use of the hospital for physicians to provide a wide range of locally available services.

—*Improved community relations:* The swing-bed program provided the hospital an opportunity to use newspapers, television, open houses, and public speaking for promotion of the program and at the same time enhanced the public's perception of the hospital.

Benefits to patients

By far the major benefit of the swing-bed program has been to the rural elderly patients, because they have been able to receive new and improved services in their communities. These benefits can be best illustrated through two case studies of typical patients in typical grantee hospitals. In these cases, the patients and families benefit from the swing-bed program because the hospitals are organized for, and hospital staff are sensitized to the special needs of, the short-stay long-term care patient.

Case Study #1

Mr. M was a swing-bed patient at Tallahatchie General Hospital in Charleston, Mississippi, a forty-five-bed hospital with a distinct part.[10] He was 76 years old when he was referred from a larger hospital's intensive-care unit, a result of an acute myocardial infarction. One week after admission to the larger hospital, Mr. M had coronary bypass surgery. Postoperatively, it was discovered that he had a cardiovascular accident during surgery. At this point Mr. M did not respond or move any part of his body. However, several days later he began moving the right side, but did not speak or respond.

The patient's family wanted to move Mr. M back home where he could receive therapy and recuperate until arrangements could be made for nursing home placement. Upon admission to the swing-bed program, Mr. M required total nursing care. The physical therapy

10. This case study was provided by Genie Goad, the swing-bed coordinator at Tallahatchie General Hospital.

department began immediately working with Mr. M three days a week with three treatments daily. Within days he began getting stronger and began recognizing familiar faces of family and staff. He started speaking and expressed how grateful he was to be "home at last." The family members were very supportive and alternated staying with the patient.

After five weeks, Mr. M was totally alert and oriented and had learned to walk with a walker with minimal assistance and could transfer himself from bed to chair. He could feed himself and enjoyed eating. Mr. M continued to have left-side paralysis, but began adapting to his disability. The discharge plan changed from nursing home placement to home health care. In the attending physician's last progress note he said, "This man has made a phenomenal recovery."

The hospital staff strongly believe that the main element of this man's recovery was the fact that he was able to return to the local hospital, the people he has known, and the town he has always called home.

This illustrates how the availability of a full range of skilled nursing services, particularly an intensive rehabilitation program, can benefit the patient in two major ways: by avoiding transfer to a nursing home outside the community, and by facilitating recovery near home where the family can be closely involved with the patient's care.

Case Study #2

Mrs. C is a 71-year-old female who had been admitted to the Scott County Hospital in Scott City, Kansas, a number of times in the past with circulatory problems.[11] During her last admission, it was also discovered that Mrs. C was diabetic. Mrs. C had no family living in Scott City.

Mrs. C was approached about nursing home care after her diabetes was discovered but she refused to consider that option. She was allowed to return to her own home with the support of the home health department. However, she had been home for only a short period before she refused to allow the health nurse into her apartment.

It was only a few weeks until Mrs. C was once again a patient in the hospital, this time with gangrene, resulting in the loss of a leg. Her amputation resulted in an admission into the swing-bed program. Staff once again began working with Mrs. C to examine the options available to her following discharge. It became more apparent to Mrs. C through her rehabilitation that she would not be able to return to her apartment.

11. This case study was provided by Jacqueline Ann John, swing-bed coordinator of Scott County Hospital.

During her swing-bed stay she was in a semiprivate room. Her roommate, Mrs. H, also was struggling with a decision to go to a nursing home. When Mrs. H moved to a nursing home, the social service designee started taking Mrs. C to the nursing home to visit Mrs. H and they sometimes stayed for a group activity.

As Mrs. C visited the nursing home, her resistance to the transfer decreased and she finally agreed to allow the director of nursing and chaplain prepare her belongings for storage. She was transferred to the nursing home, although it was clear there would be some difficulties in her adjustment. Mrs. C has returned as a patient at Scott County once since her transfer to the nursing home. She was eager to return to the nursing home as she prepared for hospital discharge.

Mrs. C is a good example of how the swing-bed program at Scott County Hospital has been a vital link for elderly people faced with the reality of no longer living independently in their own home. The program has been available to provide the needed support as patients and their families examine their alternatives and move through the difficult transition into an institutional living arrangement.

Conclusions   Although this paper has focused on the positive aspects of the demonstration, we do not intend to suggest that there are no problems with the program or its implementation. Potential problems include the viability of small rural hospitals in weak rural economies, the difficulties of attracting specialized staff such as physical therapists to isolated rural areas, the lack of funding for long-term care in rural communities, and potential gaming of the reimbursement to maximize hospital reimbursement. Problems of implementation have been discussed in detail elsewhere.[12]

Another issue that has not been addressed in this paper is the applicability of the swing-bed concept to hospitals other than small rural ones. In brief, there are no findings to indicate that this program should not be tried in larger hospitals and nonrural communities. Even in those settings where conversion to nursing home beds might be called for, there would still seem to be a place for swing beds. The incremental costs of the service seem to be low for the benefits gained, so long as any distinct part in a large hospital is fully occupied.

The data and case studies that have been presented indicate the following preliminary conclusions about the demonstration.

12. Kovner and Richardson, "Implementing Swing-Bed Services in Small Rural Hospitals."

—Swing-bed services can be implemented by most small rural hospitals without financial abuse and with cooperation of the local nursing homes.

—State hospital associations can increase the participation and success of eligible hospitals in implementing swing-bed services through promotion and development of technical assistance in close proximity to small rural hospitals.

—Swing-bed hospitals can improve patient care for acute-care as well as long-term care patients in the hospital and can provide other long-term care services within local communities.

—Swing-bed services can help the financial status and survival of small rural hospitals.

In summary, we think the demonstration will show that the swing-bed program has the potential to provide a needed service to the rural elderly while benefiting most small rural hospitals. Although it is a policy option that can work and therefore should be maintained, we do not suggest that it is a panacea for the rural elderly's long-term care needs or for the survival of all rural hospitals. The problems are too large for one limited and specific program to solve. However, we feel the swing-bed concept should remain an essential part of a national rural health policy and warrants exploration as part of a national long-term care policy.

Cost Issues

STEVEN A. FINKLER

AFTER twenty years of rising health care expenditures, cost is a key concern in any proposed modification of the way health care services are provided. An example is the current emphasis on reducing the lengths of stay in acute-care hospitals. Swing-bed programs, which propose treatment of long-term care patients in acute-care hospital beds, would result in more patient-days in acute-care hospitals. Does such an approach consume fewer resources than other available options?

This paper compares the costs of swing-bed programs with the costs of constructing and operating new nursing homes. It presents calculations of cost effectiveness and raises questions for which additional empirical evidence is needed in order to draw well-reasoned conclusions.

The basic rationale behind the assertion that swing beds are cost effective is fairly straightforward. If an acute-care hospital bed would otherwise be empty, the costs to the hospital of having a long-term care patient in that bed are the incremental operating costs incurred for the care of that patient. With a growing aged population, the number of beds needed for long-term care is increasing, and the construction cost for new nursing home beds is substantial. This paper assumes the use of swing beds when nursing homes in a geographic area are operating at capacity levels.

However, the problem is complex. Hospitals tend to have higher per diem operating costs than nursing homes. Construction costs for acute-care hospital beds are greater than for nursing home beds. More ancillary services might be provided to a long-term care patient in an acute-care hospital than that patient would receive in a skilled nursing facility. Moreover, I could find no evidence indicating whether such increases in cost and services yield improved health outcomes.

Background Palmer and Cotterill present a thorough review of studies of nursing home costs, basing much of their discussion on the prior

42

work of Bishop.[1] The range of cost-determining characteristics
they discuss includes scale of operations, provider type (profit
versus nonprofit), location, and regional differences in input costs.
Also relevant is the nature of the product, manner of payment,
certified level of care, occupancy rate, patient turnover, and source
of payment.

Scale of operations is a concern in this paper. In attempting to
estimate the cost per patient-day in a new nursing home, an
important factor would be the effect of the size of that home and
its occupancy rate on its ability to spread fixed costs. Provider
type is also an issue, to the extent that a new nursing home might
be for-profit and seek an equity return higher than that demanded
by a not-for-profit hospital. The nature of the product is a concern.
For instance, will patients receive more lab tests simply because
their bed is in an acute-care facility? Such additional testing might
reflect a higher quality of rehabilitative care, or it might simply
reflect that lab tests are cost-reimbursed for long-term care patients.

Regional differences can be ignored because both the swing-
bed usage and addition of nursing home beds would presumably
occur in the same general region. Manner and source of payment
will also be ignored; I will assume that this would be the same
for swing-bed patients as for nursing home patients. While that
may not be the case, it is not likely to have a major effect on the
costs of treating a long-term care patient in the two settings
(acute-care swing beds versus nursing homes).

It is largely accepted that the average cost for a long-term care
patient in a nursing home is less than that for a long-term care
patient in a hospital. Several recent studies found a cost difference
even between a freestanding nursing home and a hospital-based
nursing home. Schlenker and associates found that the average
total cost per day was $36.92 for their sample of thirteen hospital-
based facilities, but only $26.25 for their sample of sixty-five
freestanding nursing homes. Similarly, Sulvetta and Holahan
report average costs of $105.31 per day for hospital-based facilities
and only $61.12 for freestanding facilities. Cotterill found that
hospital-based units reported over 60 percent higher average costs
than freestanding institutions.[2]

    1. Hans C. Palmer and Philip G. Cotterill, "Studies of Nursing Home Costs," in
Ronald J. Vogel and Hans C. Palmer, eds., *Long-Term Care: Perspectives from Research and
Demonstrations* (U.S. Department of Health and Human Services, Health Care Financing
Administration, 1983), pp. 665–721; and Christine E. Bishop, "Nursing Home Cost
Studies and Reimbursement Issues," *Health Care Financing Review*, vol. 1 (Spring 1980),
pp. 47–64.
    2. Robert Schlenker, Peter Shaughnessy, and Inez Yslas, "The Effect of Case-Mix and
Quality on Cost Differences between Hospital-based and Freestanding Nursing Homes,"

Shaughnessy and associates completed a broad study evaluating eighty-two swing-bed hospitals in 1974–78.[3] They examined both incremental and full costs. All of the data came from medicare cost reports, which are of questionable usefulness. Although Shaughnessy reports that medicare cost data is audited and standardized, hospitals have had great incentives to manipulate the reporting system to maximize reimbursement.

Among the methods used in the Shaughnessy study were some of questionable usefulness, such as an approach that sought to separate hospital fixed and variable costs and then to assume that swing-bed costs could be calculated from the variable cost estimates. However, suppose that a nurse supervisor is a fixed cost and nurse staffing is variable over significant volume changes. The Shaughnessy approach applied over a period of years might pick up costs that are really step-fixed as if they were variable. Adding one swing-bed day might not change staffing costs, but adding 200 patient-days might change staffing costs, and thus they would appear variable.

However, Shaughnessy also used an incremental costing approach that is very similar in basis (although it differs in several minor specifics) to the study undertaken here. There is one difference of particular importance. Costs of nursing home care and swing-bed care appear to vary substantially between urban and rural facilities and from state to state. Previous studies show little consistency in dollar amounts estimated. Practices seem to differ substantially. This paper presents the data with a significant emphasis on sensitivity analysis. Each element of cost that is approximated is presented with a range rather than a single number. The results can be adjusted to fit appropriate assumptions for the specific circumstances in any given state or in rural versus urban settings.

Determining relevant costs   In trying to determine whether swing beds are a financially cost-effective approach, the key issue rests on a comparison of the construction and operating costs of new nursing home beds with

---

Inquiry, vol. 20 (Winter 1983), pp. 361–68; Margaret B. Sulvetta and John Holahan, "Cost and Case-Mix Differences between Hospital-based and Freestanding Nursing Homes," *Health Care Financing Review*, vol. 7 (Spring 1986), pp. 75–84; and Philip G. Cotterill, "Casemix and Cost: A Study of the Difference between the Routine Per Diem Operating Costs of Hospital-based and Free-standing SNFs" (Health Care Financing Administration, Institutional Studies Branch, April 1980).

3. Peter W. Shaughnessy and others, *An Evaluation of Swing Bed Experiments to Provide Long-Term Care in Rural Hospitals,* vol. 2 (Denver: University of Colorado Center for Health Services Research, March 1980).

the operating costs of treating the same patients in a hospital swing-bed setting.

This question is a difficult one because it is necessary to determine the costs that are relevant. Should the hospital costs be the average costs or the full costs? Is data from the medicare cost report accurate enough to be useful? Medicare cost reports suffer from a variety of weaknesses, making the data they provide somewhat suspect.[4] For example, the order of allocation used in a hospital step-down report may be optimal for maximizing reimbursement, but may not accurately reflect consumption of resources by department or patient.

It should be noted that the swing-bed concept does not presume that patients will remain hospitalized for periods when they could otherwise be discharged to their *home*. Certainly one goal of the DRG system is to create shorter lengths of stay in that fashion. Another goal of the DRG system, one might argue, is to move patients along to the least costly appropriate form of care. In many cases that calls for moving patients from acute-care facilities to long-term care facilities. However, that goal is based on the long-run perspective in which facilities are replaced over time. In the long run, if patients classified as acute-care patients could be adequately treated in a long-term care facility, there would be an overstatement of the need for acute-care beds. Presumably acute-care beds are more expensive to construct than long-term care beds. A large number of hospitals are nearing the end of their useful lifetime; thus, appropriate measurement of the need for construction of replacement beds is a vital concern.

However, swing-bed patients are not classified as acute-care patients. In calculating the economic efficiency of swing beds, I assume that additional new acute-care hospital beds will not be built for long-term care patients, but rather that existing empty beds are being used. If this is the case, and new acute-care beds would not be built to continue such treatment beyond the life of the existing acute-care facility, then the original construction cost of the acute-care hospital is not a relevant cost. Only costs that would increase, so-called incremental costs, should have a bearing on cost comparisons for alternative modes of providing care.

This relevant costing approach has not always been followed in trying to determine the relative costliness of nursing homes versus acute-care hospitals. For example, several studies have

4. Steven A. Finkler, "The Distinction between Cost and Charges," *Annals of Internal Medicine*, vol. 96 (January 1982), pp. 102–09.

indicated that acute-care stays are far more expensive than nursing homes. If the difference is great enough, it would present an argument against swing beds. However, those studies, such as the ones performed by Hall, Lefebvre and associates, and Russell, focused on average cost data.[5] As Hochstein correctly points out, because of the joint nature of much of hospital production, many hospital costs would remain unchanged if extended-care patients were removed from the hospital.[6] Therefore average cost data is misleading.

There is a paucity of empirical data on the costs of serving long-term care patients in acute-care hospitals. Hochstein provides the first published data, but the absolute amounts are in 1972 dollars. However, Hochstein's results are still of great interest. He found that long-term care patients had lab tests one-third as often and X-rays one-fourth as often as the average inpatient. One implication of this is that the additional cost of a long-term care patient is likely to be less than that of an acute-care patient. If so, not only are average costs (which include a variety of fixed costs that an additional patient would not affect) too high a measure of a long-term care patient's effect on an acute-care hospital, but even the average incremental cost per patient for the hospital is too high.

Unfortunately, however, one cannot simply determine the average incidence of lab tests, X-rays, and other ancillaries for nursing home patients and compare that result with the incidence for patients in a swing-bed program. That would tend to understate the nursing home cost, as nursing home patients are transferred to acute-care hospitals when problems arise.

A swing-bed patient in an acute-care hospital might simply receive an extra test and still be classified as a long-term care patient. A nursing home patient would be transferred to an acute-care setting to have the test performed. The associated costs of the transfer and inpatient stay would not be captured if one simply measured comparative incidence for patients in nursing homes versus swing-bed patients. Thus a study of relative consumption of ancillary services by swing-bed patients and nursing home

5. Emmett M. Hall, *Canada's National-Provincial Health Program for the 1980's* (Ottawa: Department of Health and Welfare, 1980); L. A. Lefebvre, Z. Zsigmond, and M. S. Devereaux, *A Prognosis for Hospitals: The Effects of Population Change on the Need for Hospital Space 1967–2031* (Ottawa: Statistics Canada, 1979); and Louise B. Russell, "The Impact of Extended-Care Facility Benefit on Hospital Use and Reimbursement under Medicare," *Journal of Human Resources,* vol. 8 (Winter 1973), pp. 57–72.

6. Alan Hochstein, "Treating Long-Stay Patients in Acute Hospital Beds: An Economic Diagnosis," *The Gerontologist,* vol. 25 (April 1985), pp. 161–65.

patients would have to follow nursing home patients over a period of time and include their acute-care episodes.

In some cases, use of swing beds can completely eliminate the cost of transferring a patient. One would suspect that most of the costs related to transferring patients are related to ambulance transportation. However, there is no empirical evidence. In addition to saving ambulance costs, keeping the patient in the hospital as a swing-bed patient avoids having to go through admitting, billing, and establishing a medical record twice. However, the marginal costs of these activities are likely to be minor. Although avoiding transfers is a savings generated by use of swing beds, data are inadequate to include a measure of this savings in the calculations in this paper.

Hochstein estimated that the marginal cost of a long-term care patient in an acute-care hospital is only 24–30 percent of the average cost. These figures seem reasonable in light of the above discussion and Lipscomb's survey of twenty papers, which showed that the marginal cost of treating an acute-care patient in an acute-care setting was about 40 percent of average costs.[7] Wiener has indicated that he would expect the marginal costs of a long-term care patient in an acute-care hospital to be much less than the costs estimated by Hochstein.[8]

Cost calculations

To ascertain the cost effectiveness of swing beds, a formal, rigorous study of the relevant incremental costs must be undertaken. Such a study would be both time consuming and costly, requiring a major data collection effort, because the cost information needed is not readily available from hospital and nursing home records. However, before proposing a study of such magnitude, it is worth considering on the basis of some very rough suppositions whether it is even potentially possible for the swing-bed alternative to be cost effective.

This paper will present numerical analyses to provide some basic information about the relative costs of a swing-bed program. The focus is on the per diem costs. I do not evaluate the total costs that might be higher if swing-bed patients have increased utilization, either in patient-days or ancillary services. Further, the focus is on resources consumed, rather than on payment

7. Joseph Lipscomb, Ira E. Raskin, and Joseph Eichenholz, "The Use of Marginal Cost Estimates in Hospital Cost-Containment Policy," in Michael Zubkoff, Ira E. Raskin, and Ruth S. Hanft, eds., *Hospital Cost Containment: Selected Notes for Future Policy* (New York: Prodist, 1978).

8. Personal communication from Joshua M. Wiener, March 26, 1986.

systems. Thus I made no attempt to evaluate whether there might be double payment in cases in which some swing-bed costs are already included in the DRG rate calculation for the patient's acute-care stay. The extent to which the specific numbers used are considered reasonable is subjective. Because of the roughness of much of the data, the analysis relies heavily on the use of sensitivity analysis. However, the analysis should provide some insight regarding which resources would tend to be incremental and which would not.

The comparison is between a swing-bed acute-care hospital setting, a currently existing nursing home setting, and a proposed new nursing home. To begin the analysis, one can break costs into two major categories, capital and operating.

Capital Costs

Capital costs consist of the acquisition cost of land, building, and equipment; interest incurred to finance the acquisition; and a return on equity.

For this analysis, capital costs are not considered to be relevant costs for acute-care hospitals or existing nursing homes. Swing-bed programs are applicable only where acute-care hospitals already exist and have excess capacity. Given that excess capacity, hospitals would not have to incur any additional capital costs. The same argument holds for already existing nursing homes that have excess capacity. However, capital costs are relevant for new nursing homes, because capital costs would have to be incurred in order for them to come into existence.

There has been a longstanding debate over how much, if any, return on equity (or return on investment) health care organizations are entitled to. The current theoretical leaning would be that all health care organizations, whether for profit or not for profit, need a return on equity to cope with inflation, adoption of new technologies, and expansion and replacement of buildings and equipment. On the other hand, federal policy on medicare payments has been moving away from inclusion of a specific return on investment. Hospitals with costs below the federal payment rates would however be implicitly earning a return on investment.

In any case, while there is little agreement on whether a return on equity is actually a cost, there is agreement that interest on debt should be considered a cost. Varying capital structures make it difficult to generalize about the level of equity (versus debt) that we are likely to observe for any given institution. One hospital or nursing home might finance half of its long-term assets from equity, while another might have only 10 percent equity.

In this paper I will include return on equity as a cost by calculating interest on the entire cost of acquiring and constructing new facilities, whether the source of financing is debt or equity. The interest calculated on the equity portion of the investment will serve adequately as a proxy for the return on equity. This is not likely to have a major effect in this paper, since most new nursing home construction is highly leveraged, with a very low equity component. To the extent that one believes a return on equity would be higher or lower than the interest rate on debt, an adjustment could be made in the weighted average interest rate used in the calculation.

Construction of a new nursing home obviously requires a substantial amount of investment in building and equipment that will likely result in interest costs as well. I estimate these capital costs to be $10.90 per patient-day for 1984. A range around this figure will be developed through sensitivity analysis, once the derivation of this estimate is explained.

A representative of a large for-profit nursing home chain reported a range of $28,000–$30,000 as the average construction cost for new nursing home beds, based on 1984 data.[9] Using this information, I estimated $29,000 as the cost per bed for new nursing home beds.[10] This figure, however, is the cash cost. One must also consider the interest cost on borrowed money. As discussed earlier, the interest rate will be applied uniformly regardless of whether the money was actually borrowed. If one assumes an interest rate of 12 percent and a time period of thirty years, by using present-value mortgage calculations one can determine the monthly payment required to pay off both the principal and the interest.

I also used the occupancy rate that was experienced by the nursing home chain, 90 percent, in determining how many patient-days there would be per bed per month. By dividing that into the monthly mortgage payment, one can get a capital cost per patient-day covering both the acquisition cost and the interest. Given the assumptions stated above, the capital cost per patient-day is $10.90.

9. Telephone conversation with Bill Wright of Beverly Enterprises on October 22, 1985. At the end of 1984 they owned 101,739 beds, and in 1984 they had 31.4 million patient-days. This represented a 90 percent occupancy rate. (The number of beds increased during the year.) Because of Beverly's large size, it is in some ways more representative of the national long-term care industry than any individual nursing home would be.

10. The Dodge Construction Systems cost index for 1985 shows nursing home construction costs ranging from $44–$71 per square foot. Nursing home size ranged from 15,000 to 50,000 square feet. Cost or square foot data per bed are not available from this index, which is published by McGraw-Hill Information Systems, Princeton, N.J.

I also calculated this capital cost assuming costs per bed that were 30 percent less than $29,000, 20 percent less, 10 percent less, 10 percent more, 20 percent more, and 30 percent more. Under these alternatives the capital cost per patient-day is $7.63, $8.72, $9.81, $11.99, $13.08, and $14.17, respectively.

Other variables in the calculation are the interest rate, mortgage term, and occupancy rate. I calculated the capital costs for the seven acquisition cost alternatives ($29,000 per bed, plus or minus 10 percent, 20 percent, and 30 percent), under assumptions of occupancy rates ranging from 80 to 100 percent, interest rates ranging from 8 to 16 percent, and mortgage terms of twenty to fifty years. The results indicate a range of possible capital costs per patient-day of $4.53 to $21.55. I have selected the $10.90 figure as based on a reasonable set of assumptions. If in fact the correct capital cost is higher or lower, that would make swing beds more or less attractive.

Operating Costs

The larger portion of the costs of treating long-term care patients results from operating, rather than capital, costs. Thus the question of whether swing beds save enough capital costs (by not constructing new long-term care beds) to be worthwhile is not trivial.

The principal operating costs are salary costs from: nursing; technical areas such as lab, radiology, therapy, and social work; and support areas such as administration, housekeeping, dietary, and maintenance. In addition there are nonsalary expenses such as medical and surgical supplies, laundry, raw food, pharmaceuticals, utilities, and insurance.

As part of the Robert Wood Johnson swing-bed demonstration project, data was collected on the incremental cost of swing-bed patients at a hospital in North Dakota (see table 1).[11] These data form the base for my analysis of hospitals' incremental operating costs for swing-bed patients. I use sensitivity analysis to offset the inherent problems of relying on data from one institution.

Raw food was estimated to cost an average of $5.20 per patient-day, presuming that food consumption is approximately the same for acute-care and swing-bed patients. This may not be the case, and in other areas of the country food costs might differ. Therefore I use a range of plus or minus 20 percent, producing costs of $4.16 to $6.24.

11. Data from Dale Mackenzie of Charles Bailly and Co., Fargo, N. Dak., May 28, 1985.

Table 1. *Estimates of Per Diem Costs of Hospital Swing Beds versus New Nursing Homes, under Varying Assumptions*
Dollars

	Locus of care and range of costs		
Item and cost assumption	−20 percent	Estimated value	+20 percent
	Hospital swing bed		
Capital costs	0	0	0
Operating costs			
Raw food	4.16	5.20	6.24
Laundry	1.51	1.89	2.27
Housekeeping	0.47	0.58	0.70
Operations and maintenance	0.83	1.04	1.24
Labor	8.42	10.52	12.64
Supplies	6.00	7.50	9.00
Total costs	21.39	26.73	32.09
	New nursing home		
Capital costs[a]	8.72	10.90	13.08
Operating costs	30.52	38.15	45.78
Total costs	39.24	49.05	58.86

Sources: Author's calculations based on data from Dale Mackenzie of Charles Bailly and Co., Fargo, N. Dak., May 28, 1985, and Beverly Enterprises.

a. The per diem capital costs are evaluated on the basis of a thirty-year term for financing the acquisition or construction of each bed, a 90 percent occupancy rate, and a $29,000 construction cost. The construction cost is varied by 20 percent in each direction, while the other variables are held constant. Using present value calculations, the combined payment of principal and interest each year (based on monthly compounding) on a $29,000, 12 percent, thirty-year mortgage would be $3,580 per bed. Assuming a 90 percent occupancy rate, the bed would be occupied for 90 percent of 365 days each year, or 328.5 days. Dividing the annual payment of $3,580 by the 328.5 occupied days results in a per diem capital cost of $10.90.

If the construction cost were estimated to be 20 percent higher ($34,800), the annual payments would rise, increasing the per diem capital cost to $13.08. If the construction costs were estimated to be 20 percent lower ($23,200), the per diem capital costs would be only $8.72.

Raising either the construction cost or the interest rate increases the per diem capital costs, while increasing the term of the loan or the occupancy rate decreases the per diem capital costs. For example, using a $29,000 construction cost, 90 percent occupancy, 12 percent interest rate, and fifty-year term, the annual payments would be $3,489, and the per diem capital cost would be $10.62. On the other hand, for a $29,000 construction cost, 90 percent occupancy, 8 percent interest rate, and thirty-year term, the annual payments would be $2,554, and the per diem capital cost would be $7.77.

At one extreme, assuming a construction cost of $20,300, 100 percent occupancy, 8 percent interest rate, and fifty-year term, the annual payments would be $1,655, the number of occupied days would be 365, and the cost per day ($1,655/365) would be $4.53. At the opposite extreme, assuming a construction cost of $37,700, occupancy of 80 percent, 16 percent interest rate, and twenty-year term, the annual payments would be $6,294, the number of days occupied would be 292 (365 × 80 percent), and the per diem capital costs would be $21.55. An estimate can be calculated for any combination of values for the four variables.

The laundry cost estimate was $1.89 per patient-day, exclusive of labor. This estimate is based upon a segregation of laundry department costs into labor and nonlabor, followed by a separation between costs attributable to routine service from those attributable to other cost centers. The resulting routine share of the nonlabor laundry cost was allocated to long-term care patients on a pro rata basis. A range of plus or minus 20 percent would be $1.51 to $2.27.

Housekeeping costs, calculated in a similar fashion to laundry, came to $0.58 per patient-day. A range of plus or minus 20 percent would be $0.47 to $0.70. In similar fashion, operations and maintenance came to $1.04, and a range of plus or minus 20 percent would be $0.83 to $1.24.

Additional labor costs were calculated at $10.52 per patient-day for individuals hired on an as-needed basis for patient activity and social services. A range of plus or minus 20 percent is $8.42 to $12.64. It should be noted that a strong assumption is being made here, of no additional nursing labor, which rests upon the concept that swing beds would not make up a very large proportion of the overall occupancy in an acute-care hospital.

The validity of this assumption is affected by hospital staffing patterns. If a hospital were to staff adequately for the number of licensed beds and the hospital was well below capacity, it is likely that swing-bed patients would not require extra labor. If the hospital staffed for average census, again swing-bed patients would not call for extra labor, assuming swing beds tended to be used when the hospital was below average census. If the hospital staffed for actual census, as may well be the case, the issue is less clear. On one hand, the actual census would be higher with swing-bed patients, and that might call for additional staff. On the other hand, because of the rigid nature of hospital staffing, existing staff might be able to handle extra patients. Shaughnessy found that only one hospital out of eighty-two swing-bed hospitals surveyed had hired additional staff.[12]

The most likely area in which this assumption of fixed labor costs would not hold would be nursing. Long-term care patients consume a considerable amount of nursing time. On the other hand, that time is spread over three shifts and in some cases across several different units of the hospital. If additional nursing labor was hired, it would probably be licensed practical nurses on an as-needed basis, at a cost of $5 per hour for two hours per patient-day, or roughly $10 per patient-day.[13] When the costs are aggregated, I will consider the effect that hiring additional nurses would have on the cost effectiveness of swing beds. For now, however, I will continue with the assumption of no additional nurse staffing.

In addition to the costs described above, swing-bed patients also consume routine supplies, drugs, and nursing supplies. These costs come to $7.50 in the North Dakota study. A range of plus or minus 20 percent would be $6.00 to $9.00.

Taking the North Dakota calculation in each case, the per diem incremental operating cost of a swing-bed patient is $26.73. A

12. Shaughnessy and others, *An Evaluation of Swing Bed Experiments*.
13. Estimate provided by Hila Richardson, associate program director of the Rural Hospital Program of Extended Care Services, based on her experience with rural swing-bed programs.

range of plus or minus 20 percent around this figure yields estimates of $21.38 to $32.07.

For comparison, the next step is to determine operating costs of a new nursing facility. A new facility will have to incur all of the typical fixed operating expenses of an existing nursing home, so using the average operating cost for an existing nursing home would not be unreasonable. My analysis will use $38.15 as the operating cost per bed. This figure was calculated from the annual report of the large for-profit chain.[14] To some extent, one might argue that such a chain will be more efficient and have economies of scale. Thus this figure would be an underestimate of more typical operating costs. Palmer and Cotterill reported that for-profit nursing homes tend to be significantly less costly than not-for-profit counterparts.[15] On the other hand, one could argue that there are some nonnursing costs included in this estimate (related to the company's other lines of business) and therefore the figure is too high. Offsetting this is the fact that the chain treats many patients who do not require the same level of skilled care as a swing-bed patient. That would tend to make their cost an underestimate of the cost of nursing home care equivalent to swing-bed care.

The California Department of Health Services' annual facility report showed a 1979 average nursing home cost per day (including capital) of $25. Holahan estimated the routine cost per day for nursing homes in 1980, based on medicare cost report data, at $37.26. Schlenker's estimate of nursing home costs for 1980 was $26.25. Shaughnessy's estimate of nursing home costs in 1977 was $25.70.[16]

In order for these estimates to match the nursing home chain's cost in 1984 of $42.60 per day (including capital), the nursing home industry would have had to undergo an average annual inflation rate of 11.2, 3.4, 10.2, or 7.5 percent, respectively.[17] The wide variability in the estimates for nursing home costs presents

14. Confirmed by Bill Wright and Joyce Peru of Beverly Enterprises.

15. Palmer and Cotterill, "Studies of Nursing Home Costs."

16. Howard L. Smith and Myron D. Fottler, "Costs and Cost Containment in Nursing Homes," *Health Services Research*, vol. 16 (Spring 1981), pp. 17–41; John Holahan, "State Rate Setting and the Effects on Nursing Home Costs," Working Paper 3172-05 (Washington, D.C.: Urban Institute, August 1983); Schlenker, Shaughnessy, and Yslas, "Effect of Case-Mix and Quality on Cost Differences"; and Shaughnessy and others, *An Evaluation of Swing Bed Experiments.*

17. The nursing home chain's capital cost of approximately $4.45 per day is lower than calculated in this paper, because much of their construction is not new and was built when construction costs were considerably lower.

a good reason why I have presented a range of values for each number estimated. I accept the chain's estimated operating cost of $38.15 as reasonable. A range of plus or minus 20 percent around this estimate is $30.52 to $45.78 (see table 1). An alternative to this estimate could be achieved by collecting data from medicare cost reports.[18]

Determining the operating costs for existing nursing homes with excess capacity is also of interest. Certainly these costs would be much less than for a new nursing home, because the fixed-cost infrastructure already exists. And, on the general grounds that a patient-day in a nursing home is normally less expensive than a day in an acute-care facility, one might argue reasonably that the incremental cost of a long-term care patient in a long-term care facility would be less than that of a long-term care patient in an acute-care facility.

Total Costs

I address only the costs of hospital swing beds versus new nursing homes, not those of existing nursing homes. Based on the above discussions, existing nursing homes have the lowest cost per patient-day for incremental patients. Thus one might conclude that it is probably optimal to put long-term care patients in a long-term care setting that is already existing and has excess capacity, assuming equal levels of care. In general, however, swing beds have been proposed only in those areas that do not have nursing homes with excess capacity.

My focus therefore will be on the alternatives of construction of new long-term care facilities versus the use of swing beds in acute-care hospitals. My calculations of the range of capital and operating costs yield a potential of over 3,500 estimates of the costs of the two major alternatives. In choosing the figures to use in each case, I operated on what I considered to be a "reasonable" set of assumptions. However, every number could be challenged and could fruitfully become the base for an empirical study. The purpose of this analysis was merely to raise many of the issues

18. HCFA provides nursing home payment limits, which are 112 percent of the average per diem cost. These limits, once published, can be updated with inflation indexes. For reporting periods beginning October 1, 1982, these limits for freestanding nursing homes were $49.90 (urban) and $50.87 (rural) (47 Fed. Reg. 42894 [1982]). To update these limits to June 1984, one would have to increase them by 11.6 percent, and then to get an approximate average cost for that period, deflate by 12 percent. The result would give an average nursing home cost somewhat higher than that estimated in this paper. Such medicare figures would tend to make swing beds more attractive compared with new nursing home beds.

that are important in determining the cost effectiveness of swing beds and to determine whether it is reasonable, from a financial viewpoint, to consider the swing-bed alternative.

Given my set of assumptions, a swing-bed patient-day would cost $26.73, while a new nursing home patient-day would cost $49.05.[19] This indicates that new nursing home beds are 83.5 percent more expensive than swing beds. Thus, if every component of the swing-bed cost estimate (except nursing labor) were increased by 83 percent, swing beds would still be attractive. Alternatively, if every component of the new nursing home cost estimate were decreased by 45 percent, swing beds would still be the less costly alternative. Obviously, some components in each case may be overestimated and some underestimated. But in aggregate, the results here would be reversed only if the estimates used here contain a significant and systematic bias in favor of the swing-bed alternative.

Another interesting outcome of the sensitivity analysis is that if $10 of additional nursing time per swing-bed patient-day must be added to the hospital costs, the swing-bed cost would rise to $36.73, which would still be less than the cost of a new nursing home patient-day. If all the other estimates are accurate with the exception of labor, additional labor costs per patient-day would have to exceed $22.32 in order to make swing beds less attractive than new nursing home beds.

Discrete nature of nursing home investment

An additional factor that must be considered in examining the cost effectiveness of swing beds is the lumpiness of investment in new nursing home beds. Even if new nursing home beds were less expensive on a per diem basis, that fact would be relevant only if demand were great enough to fill an average-size nursing home.

My calculations focused on the capital cost per bed for new nursing homes assuming that a large enough number of beds

19. Medicare swing-bed reimbursement rates are substantially above the marginal swing-bed rates estimated in this paper. For 1984 the range of SNF and ICF medicaid rates applicable to reimbursement under medicare ranged from a low of $20.99 (Georgia) to a high of $132.50 (Alaska), based on data from HCFA regional offices and individual state medicaid programs. However, the fact that these rates are greater than marginal costs is in no way surprising, since the rates are based on full costs, including such fixed items as administration, insurance, interest, and depreciation. In the short run, hospitals will benefit if they accept swing-bed patients at any rate above their marginal or incremental cost. In the long run, the hospitals will not be able to replace their beds unless they receive full costs. Swing beds are a short-term solution, making use of existing excess beds in acute-care hospitals. See the paper in this volume by John Holahan for a discussion of whether hospitals should be reimbursed for swing beds based on marginal or full costs.

would be built to spread fixed costs. If a community needed two or four or ten long-term care beds, a swing-bed program would become far superior. To build a very small nursing home would mean that the essential services would still exist, but would be shared by few patients. The cost per patient would be very high.

This, of course, assumes that one could not add a few extra beds to an existing nursing home. Generally nursing homes are built in specific increments (often either forty or sixty beds). These increments fit well with typical staffing patterns. Could one or two or three beds be added to an existing facility? This might be feasible, perhaps even without significant remodeling costs. Could thirty or forty beds be added? That might also be possible, but clearly not without major construction costs.

Many nursing homes are currently at capacity. Are these homes capable of adding a few additional skilled-care beds? The marginal operating costs might be expected to be very low and therefore the potential profitability high. It would be valuable to know the extent to which nursing homes at high capacity have actually added several beds. If one observed empirically that a number of nursing homes had added several beds without significant construction cost, that might well present a solution at least comparable, if not superior, to swing beds. On the other hand, if nursing homes at or near capacity have not been adding a few beds, that might indicate a discrete break in the production function for staffing, which would be a barrier preventing such an alternative approach.

Construction of additional nursing home beds for existing nursing homes presents an interesting, but analytically complex, alternative. One might well expect some administrative economies from expanding an existing nursing home, compared with building a new facility. However, it is unlikely that a nursing home would construct an additional ten or twenty beds; casual observation suggests that nursing homes do not build in those increments. That would seem to imply severe staffing diseconomies: ten to twenty beds might be enough to require additional staff on all shifts, but not be enough to fully utilize that staff.

At the other extreme, if any one hospital were considering having fifty, sixty, or eighty beds devoted to long-term care patients on any given day, the incremental analysis used for assessing hospital costs would have to be severely revised. For example, it could no longer be assumed that nursing costs would not increase. It should be noted, however, that having as many as forty swing-bed patients at a time is well outside the range normally relevant in most existing swing-bed programs.

Thus, the fewer beds needed on the average day for long-term care, the more cost effective is the swing-bed solution, and the greater the number of beds needed, the less cost effective. Shaughnessy and associates have indicated that in their evaluation of swing beds they will account specifically for the effect of this volume-cost relationship.[20] Clearly, consideration of the demand for long-term care beds is an essential element of any final determination of the appropriateness of swing beds as a solution.

Another problem that must be addressed is the lumpiness of the provision of health services. In a decision about whether to place a swing-bed patient in a 95 percent occupancy acute-care facility or a 95 percent occupancy nursing home, both of which already exist, the difference in costs would probably be minor. In both cases the patient would require nursing care and hotel-type services. Suppose, however, that by placing a group of patients in a 90 percent occupancy nursing home rather than in a 70 percent occupancy acute-care facility, the hospital were able to close down a wing completely, while the nursing home would not have to open a wing. That is, a particular unit of the hospital was nearly empty, and, by shifting the patients out, a number of fixed costs associated with running that unit could be avoided. In that case, swing-bed usage would not make sense. The savings from caring for the patients in the nursing home might be significant. Thus the assumptions one makes about what will happen when care is delivered in different ways are crucial to the results of the analysis.

Level of staff skill

Another major issue concerns the level of skill of individuals providing care. For example, suppose that a nursing home would use a practical nurse for a certain function, but the hospital would use a registered nurse for the same function. If some additional nursing time is required when swing-bed patients are present, what level of nursing care should be considered in the cost calculation?

In calculating the cost effectiveness of a swing-bed program, should one look at the cost of the actual registered nurse providing the service or the practical nurse who could provide the service? That question rests largely on the complete duties of the nurse. For example, if there are just a few swing-bed patients, they will receive some portion of the time of a nurse who is also providing a significant portion of her time to acute-care patients. It would

20. Peter W. Shaughnessy and others, *Hospital Swing Beds in the United States: Initial Findings* (Denver: University of Colorado Center for Health Services Research, November 1985), pp. II.12–II.13.

probably be inappropriate to cost out the swing-bed nursing time based on a less qualified individual. On the other hand, if there is sufficient volume in swing beds to occupy at least one nurse on each shift, one could well argue for use of a lower-cost practical nurse in the calculation.

Ancillary costs   This paper has focused on routine care costs. Although data is not available for analysis, ancillary costs should be considered. Shaughnessy and associates have hypothesized that the incremental cost of an ancillary service would be relatively minimal in swing-bed hospitals.[21] On the other hand, if ancillary usage rates are higher than they would be for the same patients in nursing homes, that hypothesis may be rejected. As mentioned earlier, Hochstein found ancillary usage for long-term care patients in acute-care hospitals to be much lower than the average utilization of acute-care hospital patients. However, there is no evidence of how nursing utilization compares with swing-bed patients' ancillary utilization.

Additionally, one must consider the case mix of swing-bed patients as compared with nursing home patients. Here again, direct data are not available. Wiener and associates found that the bulk of studies on case-mix differences between hospital-based skilled nursing care facilities and freestanding facilities indicate a more severe case mix for hospital-based facilities.[22] One might infer from that a higher severity for swing-bed patients than for nursing home patients. Furthermore, Shaughnessy and associates noted that "swing-bed patients are more frequently characterized by subacute or medically intense problems and conditions . . . than is the case for nursing home patients."[23]

Unfortunately, one does not know the relationship between the greater severity described by Wiener and Shaughnessy and increased utilization of ancillary services. Furthermore, data are unavailable on issues such as how often nursing home patients have to be discharged to a hospital to receive ancillary tests not available at the nursing home. Thus a study of ancillary usage by nursing home patients versus that of swing-bed patients might well be biased in favor of underestimating nursing home patient utilization rates.

21. Ibid., p. II.12.
22. Joshua Wiener, Korbin Liu, and George Schieber, "Casemix Differences between Hospital-Based and Freestanding Skilled Nursing Facilities: A Review of the Evidence," *Medical Care,* vol. 24 (December 1986), pp. 1173–82.
23. Shaughnessy and others, *Hospital Swing Beds in the United States,* p. V.36.

Conclusion   Based on the analysis in this paper, one can draw the following conclusions. First, it would appear that existing nursing homes with excess capacity are likely to be the most cost-effective option for long-term care patients. However, in many cases such excess capacity does not exist. Second, swing beds represent a more cost-effective alternative in the short run than building new nursing home beds.

The reader should bear in mind that the health care industry has substantial variation. Some hospitals are rural and others urban. Some are community facilities, while others are major teaching centers. Some hospitals are nearly full, while others have substantial excess capacity. The likely impact of swing-bed patients on costs should be considered in light of specific situations.

Possibly one of the most important issues is what will happen in the long run. Swing beds are conceptually most appealing when they utilize existing empty hospital beds. However, if empty hospital beds exist, filling them with swing-bed patients may generate a false signal. A 100-bed hospital that is really superfluous and should be closed may remain open because the swing-bed patients make occupancy appear reasonably high. Alternatively, a 200-bed acute-care hospital that might be more cost effective if rebuilt as a 150-bed hospital at the end of the building's useful life may be rebuilt as a 200-bed hospital if the swing-bed occupancy gives the hospital a consistently high overall occupancy rate.

Thus, while use of swing beds in a hospital to avoid new nursing home construction is probably a wise and economical use of resources, it must be realized that this is a short-term solution to the problem of taking care of the elderly and others in need of long-term care.

The interim report by Shaughnessy and colleagues indicates that their evaluation will include incremental costs, ancillary and routine care costs, and a comparison of swing-bed costs relative to nursing home costs.[24] This additional research on swing-bed costs should shed further light on this issue.

Comments by Christine E. Bishop

THE SWING-BED policy option presents an opportunity to adjust the delivery of health care at the edges: to make a small change or to not make that change, depending on which is more efficient.

24. Ibid., p. II.12.

Considering such a marginal change can illustrate some principles that are useful in considering other resource issues in health care. As one thinks about the cost issues raised here, it is important to be sure that the costs of the right options are being considered; that the costs of alternatives are being measured appropriately; and that the time frame is appropriate, so that the discounted stream of costs for alternative strategies is being compared over the long run.

Service Definition

The basic question for cost analysis is, of course, does care for long-term care patients cost more in a hospital swing bed or in a nursing home bed? The first aspect that I would like to stress is whether the services being compared are in fact the same. Are there components of the service in different settings that might make swing-bed care more efficient or cost effective for some patients and less so for others? Quality and amenity of care are the subject of another paper, but cost comparisons cannot be divorced from quality and amenity issues. Unless quality can be held constant, unless patients are really receiving the same service for the resources expended in each setting, cost per unit cannot be compared without noting service differences.

One aspect of postacute service is length of stay. Nursing home cost comparisons tend to use the patient-day as the unit of analysis. But for short-stay patients, significant resources may be used in the admissions process and in discharge activity. Long-stay care and short-stay care might usefully be considered as different services here. This could support a conclusion for cost analysis, alluded to in Finkler's paper, that short-stay care is relatively more efficient in hospital swing beds because of the costs saved in avoiding a second admission and discharge process. This would imply that swing-bed care might be worthwhile for short-stay patients, but might not be for longer-stay patients.

Another dimension of the service, and an important reason for initiating swing-bed care, is the location of the swing-bed service close to the patient's home community. Proximity to the site of care has a great deal of value to patients and families, but this value is not recognized in the reimbursement for hospital and nursing home care. Even if nursing home care were less expensive to payers, swing-bed care might still be considered worthwhile when hospitals can serve patients nearer their homes.

Cost Comparisons

If these and other service differences can be measured and accounted for, and there are clear definitions for what the health care system should provide to these patients, then the task becomes to provide these long-term care services at lowest cost. This is when cost-effectiveness analysis becomes appropriate. Costs can be reduced by making better use of available resources; and the resource that apparently is available in rural areas is underused hospital capacity. Therefore the costs of the two alternatives are the incremental cost of serving these patients in hospital beds versus the full cost of building new nursing home beds plus the care resources used for patients there. The resources that would have to be diverted from other uses to build nursing home beds can be saved if one makes use of resources already available, in the form of capital invested in hospital beds. The question becomes, which option requires fewer resources, that is, has lower opportunity costs? Such a cost analysis should not focus on dollar cost to payers or average accounting costs, although the dollar cost to various payers affects the distribution of costs and should be considered eventually. It is important to remember that accounting cost data generally do a poor job of reflecting the cost to society of diverting resources from one alternative use to another.

Finkler's analysis keeps the focus appropriately on the incremental costs of the alternatives for the most part, although it possibly overemphasizes the terms of mortgages and alternative returns on equity. The stress on financing could be misleading if it distracts from thinking about the value of nursing home construction resources if they were used for other types of capital construction today.

Another important aspect of the problem is that a portion of hospital operating costs tends to be "lumpy": overhead costs of administration, laundry, and food services are ongoing in hospitals and would not be much increased by swing-bed patients. The cost analysis suggests that even the cost of staffing a nursing unit would not be increased by these patients, because staff hours are not adjusted up or down as the census on a unit changes. The long-term care patients' only incremental costs are then their own specific food and laundry costs. The analysis itemizes these costs effectively. But it is also necessary to consider another level of lumpy costs: the cost of running a unit as a whole. If a hospital could close an entire unit in the absence of the long-term care patients, the swing bed must be seen as responsible for the quasi-fixed operating costs of the unit as a whole.

It would also be interesting to consider what cost information hospital administrators would need to determine whether they should enter the swing-bed program, specifically whether a reimbursement rate equals or exceeds actual incremental cost, and what cost information would be useful under a unified DRG system, where hospitals would be responsible for the cost of postacute care whether supplied in nursing home beds or their own swing beds.

Cost of Alternatives over Time

The comparison should also consider the time stream of costs: new construction requires an outlay of resources today, whereas use of swing beds, even as a temporary measure, can defer that new nursing home construction for a number of years, allowing resources to be used for other purposes in the interim. An analysis of discounted total cost streams for the alternatives for a given flow of patients would clarify this issue. Reimbursement systems do ask payers to pay a certain amount per day for capital, but from the point of view of social cost, the outlay was made when the facility was built and cannot be recovered. Capital costs are sunk costs: after they have been built, neither nursing home capacity nor hospital capacity can easily be shifted to activities other than taking care of patients. So the significant fact is that capacity is available in hospitals to supply care over the next decades, and it would cost $20,000 to $38,000 per bed today to build equivalent additional nursing home capacity.

Broader Alternatives

At a larger level, though, the cost analysis may not have treated all the alternatives. It is not clear what information would be needed to say where, when, and for whom swing-bed care is cost effective. Especially when care in urban areas is considered, economies of scale might argue for consolidation of hospitals and long-term care facilities into efficiently sized, fully utilized units. This could necessitate closing some hospitals in their entirety. In rural areas, it may be necessary to keep a hospital viable, through swing-bed care, in order to provide a workshop for the local physician, so that he or she will be willing to stay in practice there. But then the problem might be better attacked by increasing physician reimbursement: if the objective is to keep physicians in rural areas, it might be more effective to assure physicians a return for practicing primary, nonhospital care rather than to foster the survival of very small rural hospitals. More efficient home care for these patients might also be an alternative both to care in distant nursing homes and care in swing beds. More information is needed to design a cost-efficient future.

Comments by Donald A. Wilson

STEVEN FINKLER did an excellent job of comparing the cost of nursing home care in swing beds with that in newly constructed nursing homes. He outlined the incremental costs that swing-bed hospitals need to incur. Depending on the condition of the patient, additional nursing care may be necessary. Heavy-care patients need more staff.

An important point is that the intent of the swing-bed program is to provide access to skilled and intermediate care in rural areas. From that perspective, it certainly is an extremely cost-effective alternative for the beneficiaries and their families. Some of our hospitals in Kansas may be more than 200 miles away from the nearest skilled nursing facility bed. In making a transfer from the hospital community to the distant skilled bed, the cost to the family is significant. With swing beds, the patient does not incur the cost of transfer, nor does the family incur the cost of traveling to that alternative site. This is particularly important when one considers that two-thirds of older Kansans live in counties classified as rural.

Swing beds also affect the overall performance of the hospital. The swing-bed program has given the hospitals another product to provide to their community. It has given them the opportunity to spread some of the fixed cost and obtain another source of revenue.

Finally, the swing-bed program has demonstrated that there are some alternatives for a cost-effective inclusion in the hospital setting of other services. Primary health care is one such area that should be investigated.

Swing-Bed Reimbursement: Objectives and Options

JOHN HOLAHAN

THIS PAPER will address a number of issues that arise in developing medicare policy for the payment of care provided in swing beds. Under current policy, medicare patients are reimbursed at the prior year's average medicaid skilled nursing facility (SNF) rate in the state. Medicaid programs can establish their own payment policies. They can use the medicare approach of paying the prior-year average SNF rate or they can employ the same reimbursement policy that they apply to skilled nursing or intermediate-care patients in other facilities. The reasoning behind using the prior year's average medicaid SNF rate is that such a rate would be less than medicare rates paid to other facilities yet sufficiently high to cover the marginal cost of caring for these patients. Furthermore, by paying the rate and not facility costs, hospitals would not have the burden of filing cost reports to medicare.

Medicaid SNF rates applicable in calendar year 1984 range from $30 to $50 per day.[1] As shown in table 1, there are some exceptions above and below these rates. These rates are considerably below medicare SNF ceilings for hospital-based facilities, which averaged over $83 in 1984. Ancillary costs are paid on the basis of costs, using the traditional formula of medicare charges to total charges applied to costs. This essentially takes the ratio of medicare ancillary charges to total ancillary charges and multiplies that ratio by ancillary costs incurred by swing-bed patients.

One concern that could be raised is that the new medicare hospital prospective payment system could provide strong incentives for hospitals to "game" the swing-bed provision. The incentives would be to admit the patient and receive the diagnosis-related group (DRG) payment, then "discharge" patients as quickly as possible from the hospital and begin collecting from medicare or medicaid at the swing-bed rate, all without physically

This research was supported in part by Urban Institute general support funds.

1. Data provided by U.S. Department of Health and Human Services, Health Care Financing Administration.

Table 1. *Average Per Diem Swing-Bed Medicare Reimbursement Rates for Skilled Nursing and Intermediate-Care Facilities, Selected States, 1983*
Dollars

	Rates	
State	Skilled nursing facility	Intermediate-care facility
Alabama	30.61	30.61
Colorado	35.45	35.45
Florida	34.97	31.19
Georgia	29.99	20.99
Idaho	38.44	36.57
Illinois	32.26	29.05
Indiana	46.25	36.52
Iowa	76.59	28.50
Kansas	33.72	26.96
Kentucky	48.09	31.85
Michigan	41.36	37.24
Minnesota	53.76	43.54
Mississippi	34.78	27.12
Missouri	40.55	35.40
Montana	40.26	40.26
Nebraska	38.59	29.24
North Carolina	49.75	36.16
North Dakota	46.40	32.31
Ohio	43.23	37.42
Oregon	46.76	34.26
South Carolina	40.88	31.19
South Dakota	34.66	30.62
Tennessee	42.34	29.34
Utah	45.25	35.76
Washington	37.64	35.73
Wisconsin	46.66	38.20
Wyoming	40.12	40.12

Source: Data provided by Health Care Financing Administration, Bureau of Eligibility Reimbursement and Coverage.

moving the patient. Anecdotal evidence seems to suggest that discharges to swing beds are being carefully monitored and that abuses are not common. Whether or not this is true, it is critical to assume that this type of "gaming" is not widespread, and I will not attempt to deal with this problem.

I discuss below a number of possible objectives that medicare reimbursement policy might pursue. I limit the discussion to medicare reimbursement policy because the overwhelming majority of publicly supported patients are in fact medicare patients. I propose a number of criteria against which possible reimbursement policies might be judged. I then describe a number of policy options and assess each of these options against the criteria. These options range from very simple approaches to more complex ones. The justification for moving to more sophisticated approaches depends on the risks associated with making mistakes. At current levels of expenditures, policies that require a great deal of sophistication are probably unwarranted. However, if the intent of national policy is to make greater use of excess hospital capacity to provide postacute-care services, then careful consideration of more sophisticated policy options is probably merited.

Objectives of swing-bed reimbursement policy

There are seven objectives that reimbursement policy for swing beds might have. It is clear that some of these objectives are somewhat inconsistent with others; thus it is unlikely that any policy can be designed to meet all criteria. At this stage, it is not clear what weight to place upon several of the criteria. Thus, in analyzing alternative policy options, I merely assess how well the various options would meet each criterion.

Use of Hospital Beds for Skilled and Intermediate Care When Appropriate

Perhaps the principal objective of reimbursement policy is to encourage rural hospitals to provide SNF and ICF care to patients in need of those levels of care. To achieve this criterion, a policy would have to at least cover a hospital's average variable cost of providing nursing home care. A policy that set rates equal to or greater than average variable costs would cover the added costs of providing nursing home services to these patients and pay some share of the fixed costs of the hospital. A policy that just covered average variable costs would make no contribution to these fixed costs. A policy that paid more than average variable costs would make a contribution to these fixed costs and therefore increase the facility's profits or reduce its losses. If a policy paid less than average variable costs, it would not be worthwhile for hospitals to participate in the swing-bed program.

The conceptual problem in developing a policy based on these principles is that it is very difficult to define average variable costs. Costs that are fixed in the short run are variable in the long run. In the very short run, all or at least most costs are essentially fixed. Thus the marginal or incremental costs of providing care in SNF beds may be very low. But over a longer term, hospitals may adjust their inputs. Nurses and administrative staff may be laid off; decisions on purchases of raw food or supplies can be adjusted to reflect low occupancy; and capital renovation can be deferred. Over the longer term, payment that does not cover average total costs will not make it worthwhile for hospitals to participate in the swing-bed program. Rates must cover average total costs because in the long run all costs are essentially variable.

An exception to this occurs because of peak loading. If a hospital must be staffed to be able to provide care at, say, 70 percent occupancy because at some point during the calendar year it will have 70 percent of its acute-care beds filled, then those costs are essentially fixed. The hospital can make no downward adjustments. In that case, the marginal costs of providing care in swing beds will actually be very low even over the long term. Low rates such as average medicaid SNF rates will be sufficient to encourage hospitals to participate in the swing-bed program to a limited extent. However, such a policy will probably assure that the swing-bed program remains small, for example, two to four beds per hospital. It will be even smaller during periods when acute-care demand increases.

A policy setting rates to cover marginal costs in this sense is not likely to solve the broader public policy problem of a pressing demand for more nursing home beds and the need for beds closer to patients' homes. If the objective of the program is to meet these broader goals, then rates must be sufficient to cover such costs as additional nurses, administrative and support staff, and food and supplies. These costs are largely not sunk, and rates must be greater than or equal to variable costs in the short run or expansion will not occur. And in the long run rates must be at least equal to average total costs because, as noted above, costs that are fixed in the short run are variable in the long run. If these costs are not covered, it would be more economical to close part of the hospital.

The problem in paying average total costs in caring for patients in swing beds is that there is then no relative benefit to public programs from using swing beds versus building new nursing homes; that is, there is no advantage reaped by the payer from using existing excess capacity. Thus a policy that initially sets rates to cover average variable costs but adjusts rates over time to cover full costs would seem to meet the objective of making it worthwhile for rural hospitals to allocate some beds for swing-bed purposes and at the same time be less expensive to the medicare program than paying full average costs.

Perhaps the most direct way to accomplish this is to establish rates that in principle cover average per diem routine operating costs. While many kinds of costs are fixed in the short term, capital outlays are probably the most readily identifiable. Payments to cover capital could be phased in over, say, a ten-year period. In this way, the objective of reimbursing the full costs of efficiently operated facilities over the long term will be met; but at the same time, the medicare program will benefit from use of low marginal cost excess capacity in the short run.

Because the ultimate objective must be reimbursement of average costs including capital, the remainder of this paper will focus on average costs, that is, establishing principles consistent with long-term objectives.

Access for Heavy-Care Patients

To encourage access for heavy-care patients, the program must pay the full average variable costs of individual patients. Characteristics of patients served in swing beds vary both within and among hospitals. It is necessary to pay rates or set payment ceilings that vary with patient conditions to encourage access for heavier-care patients. Paying *rates* that are invariant with patient characteristics will discourage admission of heavier-care patients. Paying *average costs*, that is, the average costs of patients with very different characteristics, would also discourage hospitals from placing more expensive patients in swing beds.

Efficient Care Delivery

To encourage facilities to organize care delivery efficiently would require providing strong incentives for hospitals to use all resources efficiently, including decisions on matters such as staffing, wages, and capital renovation.

Incentives for High-Quality Care

Funding must be sufficient to cover the costs of necessary resources, and at the same time facilities must be rewarded for providing higher-quality services. Recent evidence suggests that nursing homes respond to cost-containment incentives by controlling costs for services most related to patient care.[2] In the provision of nursing home services, efficiency is hard to define. Both quality and efficiency are correlated with resource consumption. Reductions in resources employed in the provision of

---

2. John Holahan, "Nursing Home Reimbursement Policy: Implications for Cost Containment, Quality and Access," Working Paper 3172–12, rev. (Washington, D.C.: Urban Institute, October 1985).

patient care can in one case mean increased efficiency, but in another basically mean a change in the product provided, that is, in the quality of service rendered.

Minimal Administrative Burdens

The administrative burdens on hospitals in assessing patient characteristics, filing administrative reports, and submitting cost reports should be minimized. Similarly, the burdens on the medicare and medicaid programs in developing and updating case-mix indices and reviewing and auditing cost reports should be minimized.

Similar Treatment of Facilities

Rates or ceilings in swing-bed facilities should be similar to those for facilities treating similar kinds of patients. Rates paid for patients requiring skilled nursing services should be the same regardless of setting. This is more of a problem under arrangements paying *rates* than under those paying *costs* up to a ceiling. In cost-based systems, it is important that ceilings be comparable; however, if facilities do not incur the costs, then clearly payment rates will differ.

Uniform Patient Access

There are considerable differences in access to nursing home beds across states. These occur because differences in state reimbursement and regulatory policies toward SNFs have encouraged development of many SNF beds in some states and few in others. Eliminating these differences would imply relatively more generous rates in states where access to SNFs is currently limited and somewhat less generous rates where access is currently abundant. This is consistent with the objective of meeting patient needs for care. It assumes that where SNF beds are in abundance, access is not a problem and that development of greater capacity through swing beds is less necessary. Conversely, where patient access to SNF beds is limited, there is a greater need to provide more beds in the community.

Policy options for reimbursing nursing homes and swing beds

Policy options for paying for care in swing beds can range greatly in degree of sophistication. The benefits of moving toward more sophisticated systems obviously increase if there appears to be a growing number of swing beds. The benefits from refined systems and the costs of mistakes are more limited if the swing-bed program will remain limited to a relatively few beds in fewer than 700 rural hospitals. The policy options are: continue the current policy, reimburse retrospective costs to a ceiling (the medicare rural hospital-based SNF ceiling), reimburse retrospective costs to a case mix-adjusted ceiling, pay prospective facility-specific rates with ceilings, pay prospective case mix-adjusted rates based on the facility case-mix index, or pay patient-specific rates based on patient characteristics.

A brief overview of how these policies fare in meeting alternative policy objectives is shown in table 2.

Continue Current Policy

The current medicare reimbursement policy is essentially a flat rate based on the prior year's average medicaid SNF rate in the state. SNF patient revenues based on these rates are subtracted (carved out) from hospital costs. Medicaid programs are free to establish their own systems for paying for medicaid-certified SNF or ICF patients in swing beds. Medicaid rates therefore can potentially be very different than medicare.

This system imposes minimal administrative burdens on hospitals and very little on the medicare program. However, this policy will probably have very mixed results in achieving the objective of encouraging hospitals to participate in the swing-bed program. The problem is that medicaid SNF rates are established in very different ways in different states. Most state reimbursement systems are basically prospective, based on facility-specific costs with ceilings set anywhere from the fiftieth to the eightieth percentile of nursing home costs trended forward. State systems contain many different choices on issues such as case-mix adjustments, groupings of comparable facilities to assure homogeneity before applying ceilings, inflation adjustments, occupancy minimums, efficiency bonuses, and frequency of rebasing.

Moreover, there are wide differences across states in the way patients are certified to receive skilled nursing versus an intermediate level of care. If the state certifies relatively few patients as SNF patients, these patients are likely to be very sick and incur high costs. If a relatively high share of nursing home patients are classified at the SNF level, there will be a greater mix of patients in terms of health status characteristics and, all else being equal, lower average costs. Since reimbursement rates are basically tied to costs, differences in case mix among medicaid SNF patients will mean differences in rates.

Given all of the factors that can affect costs in any particular state, it seems highly inappropriate to base medicare reimburse-

Table 2. *Ability of Policy Options to Meet Objectives*

Policy option	Encourage access to SNF beds	Encourage access of heavy-care patients	Minimize administrative burdens	Encourage efficiency	Provide incentives for high quality	Assure equity across facilities and states
Current policy	−	−	+	+	−	−
Retrospective costs to ceiling	0	−	0	−	−	0
Retrospective costs to case mix-adjusted ceiling	0/+	0/+	−	−	−	+
Prospective facility-specific rates with ceilings	0/+	0/+	0	+	−	−
Prospective case mix-adjusted rates based on facility case-mix index	+	+	−	+	−	+
Patient-specific rates based on patient characteristics	+	+	−	+	−	+

a. + = likely positive effect; 0 = likely moderate or neutral effect; − = likely negative effect.

ment policy on average medicaid SNF rates. The resulting rates may or may not encourage the use of hospital beds for SNF and ICF care. If the medicaid SNF rates are relatively high and exceed the average costs of care in swing beds, then hospitals are likely to be very interested in providing swing-bed care. If medicaid SNF rates are less than average costs, they are unlikely to participate. If swing beds are to be used to even out peak-load problems, it would mean that the marginal costs (even over the long term) of a small swing-bed operation are indeed very low. This, however, would imply that hospitals participating in the swing-bed program will do so at a very low level. Offsetting these purely economic incentives, however, are possible hospital objectives to meet community needs even if doing so means incurring losses.

Because the rate does not vary with patient impairment, it is possible that it will exceed the average costs of serving some types of patients but not others. Therefore this system will certainly not encourage hospitals to admit heavier-care patients. It is more likely to do so in states where rates are generally high and very unlikely to do so in states where SNF rates are relatively low.

The current system should certainly encourage efficiency. The incentive structure dictates that profits can be made if costs are held down and that the hospital will incur losses from any inefficiency. The system contains the incentives existing in any flat-rate arrangement. Incentives under the current arrangement for high-quality care are probably fairly weak. The hospital can always do better by providing less. Nursing homes seem to respond to cost-containment incentives by varying the product; that is, a possible response to the flat rate is to structure the facility to provide care in such a way that incurred costs are less than the rate. If doing so eliminates waste, then efficiency is increased. If necessary staff time or services are curtailed or limited, quality can be affected. This may be less likely to occur in nonprofit hospital-based facilities than in freestanding facilities, but there is little evidence on this.

The current policy also has the weakness that facilities treating similar patients are not treated in a comparable manner. While all hospitals with swing beds within a state are treated similarly, they are not treated the same as hospital-based or freestanding facilities treating the same types of patients. Finally, the current policy would seem to result in very different access across states. In some areas, medicaid SNF rates are high and swing beds are likely to develop; in other states, rates are low and incentives to participate in the swing-bed program are much weaker. The result is likely to be very different access to swing beds and perhaps to nursing homes in general.

Reimburse Retrospective Costs to a Ceiling

The second option would pay hospitals their retrospective costs up to the rural hospital-based SNF ceiling. This is currently based on one-half of the difference between the section 223 ceilings for freestanding and hospital-based nursing homes (112 percent of mean costs adjusted for wage differences). Because there is a wage adjustment to the ceiling, the ceiling would reflect labor costs in the hospital's area. Hospitals would be reimbursed their costs if they are under the ceiling, but would be paid only at the ceiling rate if their costs exceeded the ceiling.

Payment systems that are based on facility costs require filing of cost reports and allocation of costs between routine acute care and swing beds. These should not pose major problems. Hospitals already file cost reports and this would add only marginally to their requirements. Rules for allocating costs between acute-care days and swing-bed days would have to be developed. But similar rules already exist for allocating hospital costs to different revenue centers and for allocating nursing home costs between medicaid SNF and ICF patients.

In this option, payment rates will cover average costs unless the hospital's costs are above the ceiling. This arrangement should certainly encourage all hospitals with costs below the ceilings to participate in the swing-bed program.

Because ceilings are not case mix-adjusted, there is only limited assurance that heavy-care patients will be admitted. If the average cost of serving a patient exceeds the ceiling rate, such heavy-care patients are unlikely to be admitted. If the hospital's costs are below the ceiling, the hospital will receive full reimbursement if it admits a patient who increases the hospital's average costs only if all swing-bed patients are covered by medicare or another cost-reimbursing payer. They will not receive full reimbursement if admitting a heavy-care patient increases average costs above the ceiling rate. Thus in many instances hospitals may be reluctant to cover heavy-care patients.

This type of system is also unlikely to encourage efficiency. As long as the hospital's costs are below the ceiling, it has few incentives to monitor the efficiency of its operations. On the other hand, if its costs are above the ceiling rate, then it is essentially facing a flat rate and all the incentives inherent in such arrangements.

There are greater administrative burdens in this type of system than there are under current policy. Facilities would have to file cost reports, allocating costs to swing beds and acute-care beds as appropriate. Indirect costs would be allocated to the swing-bed center. While these reporting burdens would be greater than they are under the current system, these tasks would be no greater than those borne by many nursing homes now participating in medicare. According to 1980 data, 1,395 of 3,492 nursing homes submitting cost reports had fewer than 1,000 patients during the year, an average of less than 3 per day. Medicare would also have greater administrative burdens because it would have to determine swing-bed costs and include these facilities in its rate determination process for SNFs.

This type of system encourages hospitals to increase the quality of care, or at least certainly does not discourage them from doing so. Changes in staffing or amenities that increase quality will be reimbursed as long as those cost increases do not drive the facility's average costs above the ceiling rate.

The arrangement also allows for similar rates to be paid for similar patients regardless of setting, but does not assure similar treatment. Whether or not hospitals are reimbursed at the same rate as other hospitals treating similar patients depends on whether they incur the necessary costs to do so. But since this is essentially up to the hospital, the system is permissive in this regard. The system would also assure similarity across states. Ceilings are established in a similar manner nationwide and are adjusted for wage differences across areas. It should result in higher ceilings in states where swing-bed rates are currently low and thus improve access to SNF beds. In states where access is not an issue because rates are sufficiently high, this system would probably not increase access. Thus it should tend to even out medicare patient access.

Reimburse Retrospective Costs to a Case Mix-Adjusted Ceiling

Under the third option, payments would be determined in a manner similar to the previous option except that the ceiling would be adjusted for patient case mix in the hospital's swing beds. This option assumes that a patient assessment instrument is developed sufficiently to group patients by the relative costs of meeting their care needs. Reimbursement policy would then reflect variations in care requirements. Each type of case would receive a weight reflecting its costs relative to the average. The proportion of cases of a particular type in a specific facility would be multiplied by the weight. Summing across all cases in the facility would establish an index for the facility.

In the current system for paying for SNF care, costs are arrayed after they are deflated by a wage index. Under this option, facility costs would be arrayed and deflated by both a wage index and a case-mix index, in essence making them homogeneous with respect to wage levels and case mix. Medicare would determine the ceiling for a hospital with an average case mix, say at 112 percent of the mean for freestanding facilities plus 50 percent of the difference between freestanding and hospital-based ceilings. The hospital's case-mix index would then be used to adjust its ceiling. In the current reimbursement system, that ceiling is then made facility specific by multiplying through by the wage index for the area in which the hospital is located. Under a case mix-adjusted ceiling, the ceiling rates would be adjusted for both area wage indices and the hospital's own case-mix index.

The hospital would be paid the costs that it incurs up to the case mix-adjusted ceiling. The difference between this option and the previous one is that the ceiling would reflect the case mix served in the hospital. For example, if a particular hospital had swing-bed patients requiring very intensive medical care, its ceiling would be correspondingly higher. A hospital with a swing-bed population requiring less intensive care would have a lower ceiling.

Incentives under this arrangement are similar to those under the previous approach. It should, however, assure that payment rates exceed the average costs for even more facilities. The system would essentially establish ceilings more reflective of the costs of serving the hospital's actual patient mix. If the hospital's costs are below the ceiling, they would by definition be covered. If costs are above the ceiling that is adjusted for wage differences and case mix, then it is possible that differences between costs and ceilings are due to inefficiency; such hospitals may make adjustments and reduce costs, or they simply may opt not to participate in the program.

Because ceilings are case mix-adjusted, there is a greater likelihood under this arrangement that swing beds will be willing to cover patients with relatively heavy-care needs. There is no profit incentive to take them, as there would be under a patient-related rate system. However, unlike an arrangement that does not adjust ceilings for case mix, this one offers no disincentive. This system is still a cost-based system and does not contain strong incentives for efficiency. However, by adjusting the ceiling for case mix, it is more likely to place inefficient facilities above the ceiling and force them to be efficient.

Administrative burdens under this approach are significantly greater than under any of the other proposals. Hospitals must periodically complete patient assessment instruments in order to compute a case-mix index. Furthermore, the hospital must file cost reports allocating costs to swing beds.

This type of system permits hospitals to increase the quality of care up to its ceiling. Because the ceilings are case mix-adjusted and therefore more likely to be facility specific, there is less room for major increases in staffing or amenities than under the previous arrangement. Increases in quality may result in the hospital's costs exceeding its ceiling. Hospitals where costs already exceed the case mix-adjusted ceiling may have to reduce staffing or amenities so the payment rate will exceed their average costs.

This arrangement would receive relatively high marks for equity. Hospitals treating similar types of patients will face similar ceilings and receive similar reimbursement rates. It should also result in much greater cross-state equity and encourage greater access to SNF care in states where it is currently limited.

Pay Prospective Facility-Specific Rates with Ceilings

Reimbursement rates could be based on facility costs with a ceiling that is independent of case mix. The basis for reimbursement would be the hospital's base-year cost. Hospitals' costs would be arrayed and ceilings calculated. Hospitals with costs beneath the ceiling would have their rates established by trending forward their base-year costs. Hospitals with costs above the ceiling would have the ceiling rate trended forward. Ceilings would be the same as those for rural hospital-based SNFs. The cost base upon which the prospective rates and ceilings were established could be changed annually or rebased periodically, for example, every three years.

Under this system, the hospital's reimbursement rate should reflect its own costs in the prior year. As long as the trend factor accurately reflects the changes in input prices, it should result in a system of rates that covers average costs, that is, the average costs of caring for the case mix in the facility in the style or quality level that the hospital adopted in the base year.

Incentives to take on heavier-care patients are somewhat mixed. The hospital should receive adequate reimbursement to admit patients comparable to those reflected in the base-year costs. If the facility's costs exceed the ceiling, it may have to reduce the number of heavy-care patients that it admits in order to reduce its costs below the ceiling. Furthermore, under this system, a hospital would be more limited in its ability to take on heavier-care patients, that is, to increase the severity of its case mix. In a retrospective system it would be at least partially compensated, assuming its costs were below the ceiling, if it increased its costs in order to care for heavier-care patients. With a prospectively established facility-specific rate, it would be penalized if its costs exceeded its own trended rate.

Incentives for efficiency under this arrangement are relatively strong. A facility faces what is essentially a flat rate tied to its own previous costs. If its costs are above the ceiling, the incentives for efficiency are even stronger. One complicating issue is that of rebasing, that is, changing the cost base for projecting rates. If rates are continually reestablished based on the prior year's costs, facilities may be willing to incur losses in the current year, knowing they will gain in future years because the rate will be established on a higher base. Whether this occurs is not clear. If rebasing occurs, say, every three years, there is less likelihood of incurring current-year losses to reap higher future rates.

Quality incentives under this arrangement are probably relatively weak. The incentives are to reduce outlays on staffing or amenities. Offsetting these incentives, again, is the rebasing issue. A hospital that wishes to increase the quality of its services will increase its costs this year, knowing that future rates will be higher.

The administrative burdens under this type of arrangement are greater than under current swing-bed policy but less than under systems that adjust for case mix. Hospitals would have to submit cost reports allocating costs to swing beds; no patient assessment instruments would be filed.

This type of arrangement would receive relatively poor marks in terms of equity. It would lock in hospitals to their existing cost structure. While this cost structure may reflect case mix, it may also reflect quality of care or inefficiency. Hospitals with similar mixes of patients may therefore get very different rates. Because a hospital is penalized if it exceeds its trended prospective payment rate, it is difficult to adjust cost structures over time to compensate for differences in case mix. A similar problem occurs in solving the cross-state equity and access problems.

Pay Prospective Case Mix-Adjusted Rates

Under this arrangement, each facility would receive a rate that is adjusted to reflect its case mix but is independent of its own costs. A case-mix index for the hospital would be developed in the same way as described above, but instead of using the index to establish a ceiling, it would be the basis for setting the actual rate. A base rate would be established to reimburse a facility with a case-mix index of 1.00, say, based on the weighted average costs of all facilities serving medicare SNF patients, adjusting for wage and case mix. Assume this rate amounted to $58 per day. Facilities with case-mix indices different than 1.00 would have their per diem rates adjusted. For example, a facility with a case-mix index of 1.20 would receive a per diem rate of $69.60. The hospital would receive the same per diem rate for each patient regardless of individual patient characteristics or its own costs. The case-mix index could be adjusted retroactively if the hospital's case mix changed.

Under this arrangement, the prospectively established reimbursement rate should exceed average costs in efficiently operated facilities. Unless the base rate is constrained too tightly, the rate should cover average costs. The system could have problems for heavier-care patients, even with a case mix-adjusted rate. The system would essentially establish one rate based on the facility's case mix. Once the rate is established, the hospital may not wish to admit any patient for whom it anticipates average costs higher than the rate. That is, regardless of the case mix-adjusted payment rate, some patients will be more costly than average. The hospital will always be better off by taking patients who are less severely impaired. This can be somewhat alleviated by adjusting the case-mix index retroactively if the hospital's case mix changes. If the case-mix index increases, the rate for all patients would be retroactively adjusted upward. If the case-mix index declines, the prospectively established rate would be reduced for all patients. This will deal only partially with the case-mix issue, because the retroactive adjustment is relatively indirect.

Because this is a fully prospective system in all respects other than the case-mix adjustment, it contains strong incentives for efficiency. However, at the same time, hospitals have incentives to reduce the quality of care. Employment of resources that add to quality will reduce the profitability of each patient or increase losses.

This arrangement would impose significant administrative burdens. Facilities would be required to periodically submit patient assessment forms. Cost reports would continue to be submitted. While they would not be used in setting each rate, they would be needed for monitoring the adequacy of rates and reestablishing base rates.

This system should receive high marks for equity. Facilities with comparable case mixes would receive identical reimbursement rates. This arrangement should also assure greater cross-state equity and access. Where access is low because medicare rates have been inadequate, it should ensure increased access for medicare beneficiaries. Where access is high, the system would probably have little effect, but these access increases are less necessary.

Pay Patient-Specific Rates

Under this arrangement, the hospital would receive a different rate for each type of patient, similar to the hospital DRG system. Rates would be determined through a patient classification mechanism such as resource utilization groups. Weights or relative costs for each group would be computed, and patients falling into different groups would receive different rates.

This system would have all the benefits and problems of the hospital DRG system. How well it would work clearly depends on how successful medicare is in developing a patient classification system. As with the previous arrangement, unless the base rates are set too stringently, the system should cover average costs in an efficiently operated hospital. Hospitals providing exceptionally high quality of care may also not find their costs covered. Patients should not be denied access because they require intensive medical care or other services, since the rate should fully compensate the hospital for the added cost of treatment. This system seems superior to others in assuring access for especially sick patients.

The system has very strong efficiency incentives. It is fully prospective and hospitals are at risk for any excess costs incurred because of inefficiency, provision of unnecessary care, or unmeasured case-mix severity. Similarly, hospitals can gain by increased efficiency. The implications for quality are related. Excessive quality will be penalized and reductions in quality rewarded. There is probably less room for service reductions under these arrangements than under the hospital DRG system because it is a per diem system and reductions in lengths of stay and early discharges are not an option. Quality effects, rather, are more likely to be seen in reductions in nursing time and other inputs.

The administrative burdens are also potentially great. A patient assessment instrument must be periodically completed. Cost reports probably should be filed and used to monitor the adequacy of system payments and to periodically reestablish the base for calculating rates.

Patients with similar conditions would receive the same reimbursement rate regardless of the hospital or facility in which they are served. Similarly, the system should be more equitable across states, with rates reflecting the characteristics of the patients and not the costs of individual facilities. In states where SNF rates have been low, hospitals would receive higher rates and would be encouraged to increase swing-bed participation. In states where SNF rates are high and access is not a problem, the system would probably have less of an effect.

Conclusions   There are several general conclusions one can draw from this discussion. First, the current system for reimbursing for care in swing beds should be changed. The current policy meets few objectives other than administrative simplicity. Over the long term it is unlikely to encourage substantial participation in the swing-bed program, it does not encourage access for more expensive patients, it provides no real incentives for high-quality care, and it results in paying very different rates for patients with similar characteristics.

Second, the current system should be integrated with the general medicare system for paying for nursing home care in skilled nursing facilities. This would eliminate inequities in the current approach whereby similar patients are treated very differently. Third, the ultimate objective should be to pay for the full, not marginal or variable, cost of caring for patients in an economically efficient manner. The medicare program could retain some of the savings associated with these rural hospitals' existing excess capacity, by phasing in capital cost payments over a period of time. Otherwise, medicare expenditures would be almost as great as if new facilities were built.

Other policies vary in how well they meet different objectives. Thus conclusions on their merits depend on policymakers' objectives, that is, how they weigh objectives such as access for heavy-care patients, quality of care, or efficiency. A system employing patient-related rates would do well in improving access in general if rates are sufficiently high, it would encourage access for heavy-care patients, and it would encourage hospitals to be efficient in the employment of resources devoted to patient care. A system that was retrospective with patient-related ceilings would perhaps not do quite as well in encouraging access for heavy-care patients. It would have stronger incentives for hospitals to provide higher-quality care. The problem in either of these approaches is the establishment of patient-related rates or ceilings. Without successful development of a classification instrument, it would be difficult to establish such a system for SNF care in general or for swing-bed care in particular. Even with a workable patient classification system, the administrative burdens would be substantial and policymakers would have to decide whether the improved incentives would be worth the administrative expense.

One interim approach would be to employ a proxy measure of case mix, such as the percentage of total annual patient-days in the SNF unit that are medicare-reimbursed. Recent studies prepared for the Health Care Financing Administration have shown that this percentage is related to the case mix of skilled nursing facilities and to nursing home costs.[3] Classifying facilities by their percentage of medicare patient-days as well as perhaps by whether they are hospital based or freestanding would group facilities according to case mix to a great extent. There could simply be a set of fully prospective rates for each grouping, for example, rural hospital-based facilities with more than 40 percent medicare patient-days would have their own rate; or prospective facility-specific rates could be established with ceilings that varied by urban or rural location, hospital-based or freestanding status, and percentage of medicare patient-days. Or a similar set of ceilings could be used in a retrospective cost-based system. This

3. Margaret B. Sulvetta and John Holahan, "Cost and Case-Mix Differences between Hospital-based and Freestanding Nursing Homes," *Health Care Financing Review*, vol. 7 (Spring 1986), pp. 75–84.

would be similar to the current system for reimbursing for SNF care, but with the percentage of medicare patient-days as an additional grouping category for establishing ceilings. Making case-mix adjustments based on this category could serve as a useful interim measure while a more sophisticated patient classification system is developed.

I have not addressed issues in developing policy for reimbursing for ancillary services such as physical therapy or medical supplies. The costs of these can be rather substantial, for example, $22.30 per day in hospital-based skilled nursing facilities in 1983. Current policy assures that the cost of ancillary services are covered. Thus nursing homes have no incentive to avoid patients who may have heavy requirements for ancillary services; they also have no incentive to control use of these services. The alternative is to include these services in prospective payment rates. The problem is that ancillary costs vary greatly among facilities. This means that inclusion of these costs would lead to under- or overpayments with unwarranted gains or undeserved losses. It would also create incentives to reduce the provision of these services, therefore perhaps extending lengths of stay. Given the very limited understanding of why the use of ancillary services varies, retaining current policy seems appropriate.

Comments by Robert Schlenker

JOHN HOLAHAN's paper effectively presents and analyzes several important objectives, options, and issues surrounding medicare swing-bed reimbursement policy. Since medicare currently pays for about half of the swing-bed days of care, the medicare emphasis is appropriate. I will, however, make a few additional comments about other payers at the end of this discussion.

It is important to note that current payment policy was developed for a cost-reimbursement environment. In that context, it worked very well. Most of the present drawbacks really are a consequence of the dramatic change in medicare acute-care reimbursement policy from cost reimbursement to DRG–prospective payment.

To summarize the major problems associated with the current swing-bed policy: first, routine care reimbursement, because it is based on the prior year's statewide medicaid rates, is basically a flat-rate system in each state, with rates varying widely across the country. In particular, that variation is not associated with factors such as case mix. To illustrate the range of rates, the SNF per diem rates for 1985 varied from a low of $28 in Arkansas to a high of $132 in Alaska (the highest applicable rate in the continental United States was $85 in Iowa).

The second problem is that the per diem payment for swing-bed routine care, coupled with the PPS per case payment for acute care, creates an incentive to discharge inappropriately from acute care. The tendency to respond to the incentive is perhaps greater for a hospital with swing beds than if it were discharging patients to a nursing home in the community.

The third problem with current swing-bed reimbursement policy is that ancillary services payment is based on the old cost-reimbursement method. That creates incentives, as others have mentioned, to overprovide ancillary services to swing-bed patients.

The final problem, and the one I will emphasize in the recommendations presented later, is that it does not mesh with other long-term care medicare payment policies for either free-standing or hospital-based facilities. This is particularly true for hospitals with both a distinct-part long-term care unit and a swing-bed component. In most such cases, the hospital obtains higher medicare reimbursement in its distinct-part unit, and the swing-bed component is then typically used as a "holding area" until a bed opens in the distinct-part unit.

Despite the drawbacks to the current system, that system has a major advantage: it is administratively simple. This feature was quite important in getting hospitals to participate in the program to begin with.

Turning to the reimbursement policy objectives discussed in Holahan's paper, all are important. Unfortunately, as Holahan indicates, the objectives may conflict with one another, and they cannot all be attained equally well. The two that I feel should be emphasized are access to care by heavy-care patients and consistency of swing-bed reimbursement policy with overall payment policies for long-term care and for acute care as well.

The reimbursement policy options covered by Holahan vary on three main dimensions—prospective versus retrospective payment; a facility-average versus a patient-specific rate; and finally whether case mix is incorporated in the rate determination process.

First, I feel that ancillary costs definitely should be included in some fashion—particularly physical therapy, which is currently the ancillary service most frequently used by long-term care patients.

Second, cost apportionment and cost allocation to swing-bed

care can pose major difficulties for swing-bed facilities, where physically distinct long-term care units are not present.

Third, a critical question is whether swing-bed care should be paid on the basis of marginal or full costs. Holahan concludes that ultimately total average costs per patient day must be covered. I agree with this general conclusion, but would add that although full costs should be covered, those costs should vary according to case mix and should be determined based on data from the least costly care settings for each case-mix category. The least costly care setting for many case-mix categories may well be the freestanding facility.

In terms of broader conclusions and recommendations, reimbursement policy should be viewed from both short-run and long-run perspectives. In the short run it may not be critical to change swing-bed policy. In fact, it may be wise to wait until we know more about how medicare SNF policy will evolve, for both freestanding and hospital-based facilities.

In the longer run, swing-bed payment policy should move toward the access and consistency objectives noted above. Access for heavy-care patients can be improved by incorporating case mix into the rate determination process. Consistency can be improved by merging swing-bed reimbursement policy with other long-term care and acute-care payment policies. Thus, if medicare moves toward vouchers, swing-bed care should be included in the overall voucher coverage and payment amount. If DRG-per-case payment continues for acute care, then it should be feasible to develop, at least for some conditions, per case payment methods that combine acute and long-term care; hip fracture might be an example.

If per diem payment methods continue for long-term care, then I would opt for a prospective pricing system that is patient specific and based on case mix. The "prices" should include routine and ancillary services and should cover the total cost of care (including capital and administration) in the least costly organizational setting. As noted above, the least costly setting may be the freestanding facility for most case-mix categories. However, some conditions may be effectively treated only in hospital-based settings, and in those situations prices based on the total cost of hospital-based facilities would be appropriate.

One administrative disadvantage to such an approach is that ongoing patient assessment would be required, and that is costly. However, in the long run, patient assessment and case-mix measurement are likely to be inevitable, since payment must ultimately be tied to the "product" under any rational reimbursement approach.

A final point is that this discussion has focused on medicare payment to swing-bed hospitals; other swing-bed reimbursement issues must also be considered if an integrated reimbursement approach is to be achieved. These include medicaid swing-bed policies and physician reimbursement for swing-bed care under both medicare and medicaid. Policies affecting or affected by private-pay patients are also important, since about half of all swing-bed patients are in this payment category. Unfortunately, this discussion cannot address these important issues, but many of the general principles surrounding medicare reimbursement of swing-bed hospitals apply as well to other payers and providers in the swing-bed arena.

Comments by Kenneth Moore

JOHN HOLAHAN'S paper deals with several policy options for reimbursing nursing homes and swing beds in the future.

Continue current policy: Although the current policy seems to be working in locales where the reimbursement is high enough for the hospitals to survive, I see it as inappropriate due to the lack of consistency in the policy as it currently stands. If current policy were to be continued in the future, ancillary service costs should continue to be paid on a cost-based formula.

Retrospective costs to a ceiling: Although I am in agreement with this method for reimbursement of swing beds, this is a somewhat bureaucratic process for determining payment rates. Capital should be paid separately under this proposal and attention should be given to the long-term effect on heavy-care patients. This type of reimbursement system would not encourage improvements in the quality of care rendered to residents.

Retrospective costs to a case mix-adjusted ceiling: The problem with this type of payment process is that the administrative burden is far from simple, which could create some problems in terms of acceptance, unless case-mix information is already in place for swing-bed patients. If case-mix information was available, and if there was an allowance for passthrough of capital, this could be a very good system.

Prospective facility-specific rates with ceilings: This methodology for reimbursement would be an acceptable alternative. In order to allow for the care of heavy-care patients, a provision for a cost outlier would be appropriate with this particular payment method.

The issue of changing the cost base for projecting the rates might create problems over time. The issue of quality incentives is probably not a problem. The administrative and bureaucratic requirements under this methodology would have to be seriously considered in order to keep a simple and easily run program in operation.

Prospective case mix-adjusted rates: This payment method, along with the preceding option, ranks high as being a suitable alter-native. This method is in keeping with the currently used system and affords good predictability. It would be important for the case-mix information to be easily and accurately obtained. If not, it could be an overly burdensome process for hospitals. This approach provides good incentives for efficiency over the long term, but I would be concerned about potential gaming. Questions about quality of care would be important to monitor and control under this system.

Patient-specific rates: This method would also be acceptable to me as long as appropriate weighting factors could be determined for each group. As mentioned in the paper, it would be important to make sure the base rates are not initially set restrictively. Quality would need to be monitored and maintained over time.

In simplistic terms, any policy establishing a new reimbursement method for the swing-bed program needs to meet several criteria in order to ensure the continued success of the program. As stressed earlier, administrative simplicity is going to be integral to the success of any ongoing program. Swing-bed reimbursement and policy should be consistent with normal hospital accounting policies. Any successful program must allow hospitals participating in a swing-bed program to cover the costs of the program. However, a caution must be added that the reimbursement method cannot make the swing-bed program overly expensive so that nursing home care would seem an equally affordable alternative. The issue of capital needs to be addressed in all of the methods, as that is an important aspect of a long-term program. A balance must be maintained to assure access, quality, efficiency, and equity in programs as they are established on a nationwide basis.

Access and Case-Mix Patterns

PETER W. SHAUGHNESSY

DURING the past three decades, concerns regarding adequate access to health and medical care have given rise to a variety of health care policies and initiatives.[1] Most far reaching among such initiatives have been the medicare and medicaid programs. Targeted primarily at reducing financial barriers to needed health care services for the elderly and those in lower-income groups, medicare and medicaid have also provided a broad rubric under which a number of specific access problems have been addressed or at least raised to a level of informed debate.

The national swing-bed program is an example of a medicare- and medicaid-sponsored initiative that addresses a specific set of access issues affecting a specific beneficiary population. During the early 1970s in Utah, Bruce Walter, then the director of the Utah Division of Health, was concerned about inadequate access to long-term care services on the part of rural residents, especially the elderly.[2] He argued that the problem would be alleviated most cost effectively by allowing rural hospitals to provide long-term care in empty acute-care beds. As a result, a demonstration program was launched in twenty-five small rural hospitals in Utah, with both medicare and medicaid reimbursing for long-term care provided in acute-care beds, later termed swing beds.[3]

The data discussed in the paper were collected under Health Care Financing Administration contracts SSA-PMB-74-388, SSA-600-77-0051, and HCFA-500-83-0051. This paper has benefited from the comments of Herbert Silverman and Robert Schlenker.

1. Lu Ann Aday, Gretchen V. Fleming, and Ronald Andersen, *Access to Medical Care in the U.S.: Who Has It, Who Doesn't* (Chicago: Pluribus Press, 1984).

2. Kent M. Aland and Bruce A. Walter, "Hospitals in Utah Reduce Costs, Improve Use of Facilities," *Hospitals,* vol. 52 (March 16, 1978), p. 85; Bruce A. Walter, Donald West, and Mark D. Elggren, "Small Hospitals Find Swing Beds Profitable," *Forum,* vol. 4 (June 1980), pp. 16–17; and Robert D. Burton, "Swing-Bed Concept in Utah: A Decade of Expansion 1982," *Journal of Patient Account Management* (April–May 1982), pp. 10–16.

3. Peter W. Shaughnessy and others, *A Swing-Bed Experiment to Provide Long-Term Care in Rural Hospitals in Utah,* vols. 1 and 2 (Denver: University of Colorado Center for Health Services Research, July 1978).

86

The Health Care Financing Administration (HCFA) later expanded the demonstration program to Texas, Iowa, and South Dakota to further examine the cost effectiveness of the approach.[4]

In the mid-1980s, with a rural swing-bed program now in effect throughout the country, an additional concern related to access has surfaced. In view of the incentives to discharge patients sooner from acute care under medicare's prospective payment system (PPS), it has been conjectured that the present nursing home delivery system is inadequate to meet the needs of postacute patients who require more intense medical care than similar patients in the past, before PPS. Given the stronger medical care orientation of hospitals, such patients are more likely to receive needed medical services in hospital swing beds than in nursing home beds. It follows that enhanced access for this type of "heavy care" patient due to the availability of swing beds would be reflected in a more medically intense case-mix profile for swing-bed patients than for community nursing home patients.

Definitions and hypotheses

For purposes of this paper, a health care consumer is defined to have access to a particular type of health care if such care is both available and adequate when needed. Considered in this context, access has two components, availability and adequacy, that respectively translate into use (or potential use) and quality (or perceived quality). Traditional barriers to access include age, geographic location or distance, health status, payer source, insurance coverage, and income.[5]

Access can be considered in an absolute or a relative sense. The above definition refers to access in an absolute sense in that it states that the necessary care is available and adequate whenever needed. Because this is a difficult definition to work with pragmatically, it is more useful to refer to relative access. The principle of relative access states that a consumer has access to care if such care is *as* available and *as* adequate for this consumer as it is for other consumers. At times it is appropriate to restrict the com-

4. Peter W. Shaughnessy and others, *An Evaluation of Swing Bed Experiments to Provide Long-Term Care in Rural Hospitals*, vols. 1 and 2 (Denver: University of Colorado Center for Health Services Research, March 1980); and Peter W. Shaughnessy and Eileen A. Tynan, "The Use of Swing Beds in Rural Hospitals," *Inquiry*, vol. 22 (Fall 1985), pp. 303–15.

5. Aday, Fleming, and Andersen, *Access to Medical Care in the U.S.*; Karen Davis and others, "Access to Health Care for the Poor: Does the Gap Remain?" *Annual Review of Public Health*, vol. 2 (1981), pp. 159–82; Victoria D. Weisfeld, ed., *Updated Report on Access to Health Care for the American People* (Princeton, N.J.: Robert Wood Johnson Foundation, 1983); and Gail Wilensky and Marc L. Berk, "Health Care, the Poor and the Role of Medicaid," *Health Affairs*, vol. 1 (Fall 1982), pp. 93–101.

parison group of other consumers to a particular subgroup into which the consumer of interest falls, such as the elderly if one is comparing access to long-term care for the elderly at one time relative to another time.

Measures of the availability of access typically involve use, use rates, or specific dimensions of use such as case mix or other patient characteristics. Adequacy is less frequently considered a component of access because the tacit assumption is made that adequate services are provided. Nonetheless, a comprehensive assessment of access would entail adequacy measured in terms of patient outcomes, structural or process indicators of quality, or patient satisfaction.

The primary focus in this paper is on relative access, which is examined using case mix, other patient attributes, and certain measures of use. Thus the availability dimension rather than the adequacy dimension is of primary concern. Since case mix is a critical construct in the sequel, it is appropriate to distinguish between case mix and both service mix and patient mix, which are also considered, but to a lesser extent.[6] In view of the focus on relative access, my empirical approach deals with comparisons, usually involving rural swing-bed patients and rural nursing home patients.

My access hypotheses are:

—Long-term care patients with more intense medical care needs in rural areas have improved access to such care under the swing-bed program. This hypothesis is tested by comparing medical care needs reflected by the case-mix and service-mix profiles of swing-bed patients with those of nursing home patients in similar communities. The use of service-mix variables must be qualified

6. *Case mix* refers to a group of patients and is defined in terms of aggregated health status variables that are physiologically or psychologically intrinsic to the individual and determine or mitigate his health care needs. Variables such as age, sex, ability to dress one's self, degree of incontinence, cognitive impairment, and the presence of a surgical wound are health status variables that, when aggregated over a specified patient group, can be used to measure the case mix of the group.

Service mix also refers to a group of patients, but is defined in terms of aggregated health services extrinsic to the individual that are provided in response to his health care needs. Variables such as the number or provision of lab tests, physician visits, bathing care, indwelling catheter, wound care, physical therapy, and medications are service variables that, when aggregated across patients, can be used to measure the service mix of a patient group.

Other patient characteristics such as payer source, home situation, marital status, and distance to residence are often important in use or access analyses, but are neither case-mix nor service-mix variables. For convenience, they are referred to as *patient-mix variables* in this paper.

in this regard, since it rests on the assumption that services are provided appropriately, in accord with patient needs.

—Owing to the case-mix differences postulated above, competition between swing-bed hospitals and comparison nursing homes is expected to be inconsequential in most communities. Changes in the occupancy rates of community nursing homes in one state and the reaction of community nursing home administrators in several states are used to test this hypothesis.

—Elderly long-term care patients in rural communities are more likely to receive care in their home community if swing beds are available than if they are not. This community retention hypothesis is tested by (a) comparing the proportion of institutional long-term care patients receiving care in their home community before and after the presence of swing beds and (b) comparing the distance traveled from home for swing-bed patients and community nursing home patients.

Data and methods

The major data set used to test the above hypotheses was obtained as part of an ongoing evaluation of the national swing-bed program. Data collection involved cross-sectional random samples of long-term care patients in thirty-three rural swing-bed hospitals and forty nursing homes during 1984 and 1985. Most nursing homes were within fifty miles of swing-bed hospitals, although a few were slightly more distant. The swing-bed hospitals were from twelve states, and the nursing homes were from ten of the twelve states. Nursing homes were selected from communities relatively similar to swing-bed communities in terms of population density and absence of a highly urbanized area. All swing-bed hospitals and most nursing homes were certified for skilled nursing facility (SNF) care. Some of the nursing homes cared only for intermediate-care facility (ICF) patients, but were selected because they were the only facilities in swing-bed communities or because there were relatively few SNF beds in the selected communities. If such ICF facilities had been excluded, it would have rendered invalid the comparison of the case mix in swing-bed hospitals to the case mix of nursing homes in swing-bed communities or similar rural communities.[7]

7. The samples were selected randomly during 1984 and early 1985, without regard to level of care or payer source, since the primary objective of the analysis was to compare rural swing-bed patients with rural nursing home patients. The study design called for sampling with replacement. Although the samples were cross sectional as opposed to longitudinal, patients were selected from the same facilities at several different points in time because only a few long-term care patients occupied hospital swing beds at any single

Fourteen categories of variables were used in the case-mix, service-mix, and patient-mix analyses. Case-mix variables were divided into prevalence indicators, severity indicators, indicators of primary or secondary diagnosis, disability and problem scales, and certain aggregate indicators. More complete descriptions of the variables and information on sampling and statistical methods is given elsewhere.[8]

As part of the evaluation of the South Dakota swing-bed experiment in the 1970s, nursing home occupancy rates were obtained from the Department of Health in South Dakota. These data were used to compare occupancy rates in rural nursing homes before and after the implementation of the experimental swing-bed program in that state. In order to assess the potential for swing-bed care substituting for (that is, competing with) nursing home care, data were analyzed from surveys of 161 nursing home administrators conducted during the demonstrations in the late 1970s in Texas, Iowa, and South Dakota.

Medicare claims data were analyzed to examine variations in the percentage of rural residents receiving SNF care in rural and urban communities before and after the implementation of the experimental swing-bed approach in Utah. To examine the community retention issue, data were used from surveys of thirty-three swing-bed physicians, thirty-one swing-bed nurses, and thirty-four nurses at community nursing homes in twelve states in 1985. The key question was the extent to which these nurses and physicians felt long-term care patients were being treated more often in their home communities as a result of the swing-bed program.

Findings

Table 1 presents differences between 552 swing-bed patients and 540 nursing home patients for selected variables from the fourteen

---

time. The same sampling procedures were used in nursing homes in order to obtain approximately the same number of patients at each time point for purposes of controlling for seasonal case-mix trends over a period of several months.

Thus, an individual patient was eligible to be selected for the sample at more than one time point. The number of swing-bed patients who appeared more than once in the sample was greater than the corresponding number of nursing home patients, owing to the smaller total sampling frame (that is, census at the time of data collection) for swing-bed hospitals. To assess the degree to which this influenced final results, comparisons were conducted using unduplicated patient observations. The same general patterns and trends occurred for these analyses as for the more appropriate analyses that allowed for duplication of the same patients at different time points. Further information on reliability, data collection instruments, sampling, and data collection procedures is available in Peter W. Shaughnessy and others, *Hospital Swing Beds in the United States: Initial Findings* (Denver: University of Colorado Center for Health Services Research, November 1985).

8. Ibid.

categories. Other important differences for variables not included in table 1 are highlighted in the discussion below. All statistically significant differences are discussed in detail elsewhere.[9]

The Medical Intensity of Case Mix and Service Mix

The rehabilitation potential of swing-bed patients was generally regarded as better than that for nursing home patients. Over 50 percent of the swing-bed patients' rehabilitation potential was judged as good or moderate and 25 percent judged as good, contrasting substantially with 21 percent and 3 percent, respectively, for nursing home patients. In addition, a substantially higher proportion of swing-bed patients had been in the facility for less than thirty days: 56 percent versus only 8 percent among nursing home patients. The hypothesized subacute orientation of swing-bed hospitals is further substantiated by the finding that a greater proportion of those patients required the skilled nursing level of care (60 percent versus 37 percent). This variable is somewhat problematic in that it uses level of care as determined by the provider. Although the definition of SNF level of care varies from state to state and is even subject to discrepancies from facility to facility, the magnitude of the difference suggests a stronger orientation toward skilled nursing care in swing-bed hospitals than in community nursing homes.

There was also a substantial discrepancy in medicare and medicaid days between swing-bed hospitals and community nursing homes. Medicare covers a significantly greater proportion of long-term care days in swing-bed hospitals (46 percent) than in community nursing homes (9 percent). In fact, the medicare figure for community nursing homes in rural swing-bed communities is slightly higher than the national average, which is closer to 2 percent. On the other hand, medicaid, which is the dominant payer for nursing homes throughout the country, is in fact the dominant payer for rural nursing homes in swing-bed communities (55 percent), but pays for only a small portion (7 percent) of swing-bed days. The percentage of days covered by other payers, almost exclusively private pay, is relatively comparable in the two facilities (47 percent in swing beds versus 36 percent in nursing homes). The involvement of private pay is further evident from the fact that the vast majority (86 percent) of ICF swing-bed days are private pay days.

Nursing home patients tend to be more functionally disabled, as indicated by the next category of variables. These deal with

9. Ibid.

Table 1. *Characteristics of Long-Term Care Patients in Swing-Bed Hospitals and Nursing Homes, 1984 and 1985*[a]
Percent unless otherwise indicated

Characteristic	Mean for swing-bed hospital patients[b]	Mean for nursing home patients[b]
General		
Age (years)	81.2*	81.4*
Distance to residence (miles)	20.8**	49.9**
Married	29.4	17.3
Skilled nursing care classification	60.1	37.3
Admitted from acute care	75.9	50.8
Good to moderate rehabilitation potential	54.3	21.1
Current stay less than 30 days	55.6	8.1
Medicare primary payer	46.4	8.7
Disability in activities of daily living		
Bathing	62.7**	69.1**
Dressing	60.1**	66.2**
Grooming	57.6	74.8
Disability in instrumental activities of daily living		
Communication	14.7	25.2
Finances	58.8	72.5
Housekeeping	71.4**	79.5**
Laundry	75.6	83.7
Administering medications	60.1	84.2
Preparing meals	65.7	78.2
Telephone	30.8	42.4
Medical or nursing problems		
Shortness of breath	20.5	10.6
Recovery from surgery	13.2	3.4
Intravenous catheter	6.3	0.6
Ostomy	2.9*	1.1*
Recent myocardial infarction with congestive heart failure	1.6*	0.4*
Catheter	20.9	9.3
Hip fracture in last 6 weeks	6.7	1.3
Stroke in last 6 months	7.3	2.7
End stage disease	9.0	1.8
Urinary incontinence	34.0	48.1
Urinary tract infection	10.7	3.7
Bowel incontinence	29.0	41.3
Mental status problems	40.3	58.9
Sociopathic behavior	8.4	18.3
Wandering behavior	6.9**	10.6**
Aggregate indicators (number per patient)		
Subacute medical or nursing problems	1.17	0.67
Severe subacute medical or nursing problems	0.54	0.25
Typical long-term care problems	1.67	2.54
Intense typical long-term care problems	0.93	1.57

Table 1 (continued)

Characteristic	Mean for swing-bed hospital patients[b]	Mean for nursing home patients[b]
Utilization of services		
Lab tests in past week (number per patient)	1.37	0.26
Physician visits in past week (number per patient)	2.84	0.32
X-rays in past week (number per patient)	0.22	0.02
Antibiotics for urinary tract infection	5.3	1.5
Intravenous medications	4.7	0.0

Source: Peter W. Shaughnessy and others, *Hospital Swing Beds in the United States: Initial Findings* (Denver: University of Colorado Center for Health Services Research, November 1985), pp. V.11–V.15.
*Significant between the 0.05 and 0.10 levels.
**Significant between the 0.001 and 0.05 levels.
a. Based on a sample of 552 patients in thirty-three swing-bed hospitals and 540 patients in forty nursing homes.
b. Unless otherwise indicated, all variables shown had a significance level of less than 0.001, determined through the chi-square test, Fisher's exact test, or Wilcoxon two-sample rank sum test, as appropriate in view of the measurement scale and probability distribution of the variable.

the percentage of patients with disabilities in the activities of daily living (ADL). They include traditional ADLs, such as bathing, dressing, and grooming; instrumental ADLs (IADL), such as communication and housekeeping; and severe ADL disabilities. In terms of the traditional physical ADLs, there is a tendency for swing-bed patients to be less dependent than nursing home patients. This parallels prior studies comparing hospital-based nursing home patients with freestanding nursing home patients, where the general conclusion was reached that a more subacute case mix typically means less dependency in traditional ADLs.[10] This finding is further reinforced by a uniform pattern of less dependence among swing-bed patients in IADLs, which usually require a greater integration of cognitive and physical functioning. And severe ADL disabilities are also less prevalent among swing-bed patients.

Another category of variables deals with the prevalence of medical and nursing problems. Patients in swing-bed hospitals have a greater prevalence of the more medically oriented problems, such as shortness of breath, recovery from surgery, intravenous catheters, and ostomies, than do nursing home patients. Although the percentage of patients who had a recent myocardial infarction with congestive heart failure were relatively few, they occurred significantly more often in swing-bed hospitals than in nursing homes. The hip fracture and stroke variables both exhibit the

10. Peter W. Shaughnessy and others, "Nursing Home Case-Mix Differences between Medicare and Non-Medicare, and between Hospital-Based and Freestanding Patients," *Inquiry*, vol. 22 (Summer 1985), pp. 162–77.

hypothesized patterns of (a) a greater proportion of swing-bed patients with hip fractures or strokes within the last six weeks or six months than nursing home patients and (b) a lower proportion of swing-bed patients with hip fractures or strokes more than six weeks ago or six months ago than nursing home patients.

The more typical long-term care case-mix indicators that deal with incontinence, cognitive functioning, and psychosocial problems exhibit a reverse trend. Higher proportions of nursing home patients had these types of problems than did swing-bed patients. A higher proportion of swing-bed patients had urinary tract infections than nursing home patients. Even among catheterized patients the prevalence of urinary tract infections remained significantly greater in swing-bed hospitals. This may be due to either inferior care in the prevention of such infections or a greater predisposition of certain types of swing-bed patients to them. For example, surgical patients and terminally ill patients, both of whom are more prevalent in swing-bed hospitals, would have a greater predisposition. Hospitalized patients in general are exposed not only to more bacteria, but to bacteria that are probably more foreign to the patient's body and therefore more pathogenic than bacteria encountered in a nursing home. Further, the manner in which the urinary tract infection variable is defined required that the condition be documented by a urinalysis or culture within the last week. Swing-bed patients tended to receive considerably more lab tests than nursing home patients. Since lab tests are done more frequently and sooner after symptoms develop, it is possible that infections are reported at a higher rate in swing-bed hospitals than in nursing homes, where more subclinical or low-grade infections may be neither tested nor treated.

Severe medical or nursing problems generally exhibit the same trend as the prevalence variables just discussed, with the exception that a slightly higher proportion of swing-bed patients exhibit depressive symptoms (14.4 percent versus 10.3 percent). This may be attributable to the reactive depression that occurs following sudden traumatic events such as a stroke or surgery, both of which are significantly more frequent among swing-bed patients.

Three categories of variables that deal with diagnoses (primary, secondary, and primary and secondary combined) tend to support the trends noted above. Diagnoses such as fracture, major surgery, and neoplasms occur with higher relative frequency in swing-bed patients, while mental disorders, circulatory problems, and nervous system disorders occur with greater relative frequency in nursing home patients. The primary or secondary diagnosis of stroke is more frequent among nursing home patients, very likely due to the phenomenon noted under the medical or nursing problem category, which indicated that a substantially higher proportion of patients with strokes occurring more than six months ago were in nursing homes. It is possible that several of the patients with a primary or secondary diagnosis of circulatory problems were also stroke patients. In any event, the greater prevalence of circulatory problems among nursing home patients is probably due to past strokes or cerebrovascular or generalized arteriosclerosis.

Three categories of variables were assigned scales: the ADL, IADL, and medical or nursing problems. They further substantiate the pattern of a more subacute profile for swing-bed patients. This is also true for four aggregate indicators. The first two indicate that the number of subacute and severe subacute medical or nursing problems is significantly higher among swing-bed patients than nursing home patients. Conversely, the number of typical long-term care problems, both in prevalence and in more intense levels, is greater among nursing home patients than swing-bed patients.

Service-mix variables point to a more pronounced pattern of utilization of medical services by swing-bed patients. This may be due to the incentives for swing-bed hospitals to receive reimbursement for ancillary services under the current cost-based reimbursement policies. From the perspective of medical care, however, the pattern suggests a stronger intensity in medical needs of swing-bed patients, assuming services are not over-provided. The number of physician visits is markedly higher for swing-bed patients. This is consistent with physicians' contentions that one of the benefits of the swing-bed approach is the oppor-tunity to visit patients more frequently. Since physicians are reimbursed for visits to swing-bed patients in the same manner as visits to nursing home patients, it is likely that many of the physician visits to swing-bed patients are not reimbursed.

To assess whether the observed pattern of more intense medical and nursing needs of swing-bed patients might be due only to the greater proportion of skilled nursing patients in swing beds, the same analysis was conducted using only SNF patients. This stratification rendered the case-mix comparisons considerably more homogeneous. With these qualifications, however, the results of the second set of analyses substantiated the overall pattern of greater medical intensity and skilled nursing needs on the part of swing-bed patients.

Competition with Nursing Homes

In the demonstration states participating in the swing-bed experiment in the 1970s, long-term care utilization in rural areas generally increased on a per capita basis during the period the swing-bed program was in place. Using South Dakota, the state with the most swing-bed days, as an illustration, long-term care days per medicare enrollee increased in demonstration project counties by 3 percent. A slight increase in the occupancy of existing rural nursing homes from 95 percent to 97 percent, the addition of forty-one new rural nursing home beds, and the provision of long-term care by swing-bed hospitals accounted for this increase. The overall increase in long-term care utilization in the rural swing-bed counties and the fact that rural nursing home occupancy rates appear to have been unaffected by the availability of hospital swing beds indicate that virtually no substitution of swing-bed care for nursing home care took place as a result of the experiments.

Of the 161 nursing home administrators surveyed as part of the evaluation of the swing-bed demonstration in Texas, Iowa, and South Dakota, 60 percent felt that a national swing-bed program should be implemented. Support for the program varied by state, however. Nursing home administrators in the central Iowa demonstration project were most receptive to a national swing-bed program, with 74 percent favoring a national program, compared with 57 percent in western Iowa and South Dakota and 42 percent in Texas. Nonetheless, the empirical evidence to date does not demonstrate any substantial degree of decreased utilization of nursing homes caused by the presence of swing-bed hospitals. Rather, as discussed further below, it appears that utilization of long-term care services available in rural communities increases because of a shift from rural residents' use of urban facilities to use of facilities in their home community. This lack of competition or substitution between nursing homes and swing-bed hospitals in rural areas also appears to be a function of an unmet need for institutional long-term care in rural communities. In rural Utah, for example, the utilization of medicare SNF care rose from 188 medicare skilled nursing patient-days to 283 days per 1,000 enrollees between 1971 and 1975, the periods before and after the Utah swing-bed experiment. Additional information on this issue is currently being gathered at the national level.

Community Retention

The analysis of medicare utilization by rural residents of Utah revealed that in 1971, 64 percent of the rural residents receiving medicare skilled nursing care were admitted to urban SNFs, a figure that dropped to less than 21 percent by 1975. Although some of this decrease was due to a decline in medicare-certified SNF beds in urban Utah during these years, the decline was not proportionate to the increase in community retention for rural areas. The decrease in utilization of urban SNFs is also reflected in a reduction in medicare SNF days provided by urban SNFs. By 1975, almost 70 percent of medicare SNF admissions for rural residents in Utah were to swing-bed hospitals.

Based on survey data from thirty-one swing-bed hospitals and thirty-four nursing homes in twelve states in 1985, 93 percent of the swing-bed nurses responding felt more patients were receiving long-term care in their home community in 1985 than in 1982. Of the nurses responding from community nursing homes located in or near swing-bed communities, 65 percent felt more patients were receiving long-term care in their home community in 1985 than in 1982. Over 80 percent of the nurses who felt community retention had increased indicated that the increase was more than 20 percent. Analogously, of the thirty-three swing-bed physicians surveyed, 97 percent felt more patients were receiving long-term care in their home community in 1985. Of these, 53 percent felt the retention had increased by more than 20 percent. Further, 64 percent of the responding physicians felt the swing-bed program had a discernible impact on retention of long-term care residents in communities adjacent to the swing-bed community.

Both physicians and nurses reported that the types of long-term care patients more likely to remain in their home community after implementation of swing beds were those with fractures, elderly who could not care for themselves, those with strokes, postsurgical patients, and cancer patients.

The primary data set indicates that the average distance to the patient's residence was approximately twenty-one miles for swing-bed patients and fifty miles for nursing home patients. Since this comparison excludes rural nursing home patients receiving care in urban facilities, it underestimates the difference in distance and travel time for nursing home patients and swing-bed patients.

Approximately 75 percent of all swing-bed patients were admitted from acute care, with about two-thirds of these, or over 50 percent of the total, admitted from the acute-care portion of the hospital itself. For nursing home patients, about 50 percent were admitted from acute care, and only 7 percent were admitted from the same facility (the hospital-based portion of a facility whose hospital-based distinct part was included as a comparison nursing home; there were seven such hospital-based nursing homes in the sample).

Conclusions and discussion

The empirical findings strongly suggest that access to institutional long-term care services for residents of rural communities has been increased by the availability of hospital swing beds. Three specific conclusions follow from testing the hypotheses.

—In rural areas, long-term care patients with more intense medical needs have greater accessibility to needed services in communities where there are swing-bed hospitals. Such patients are likely to benefit from the acute-care orientation of the medical, nursing, and ancillary service capability of the hospital environment.

—The question of whether increased access to institutional long-term care in swing-bed communities is bringing about significant competition between swing-bed hospitals and community nursing homes cannot be definitively answered at this time. Although a substantial minority of nursing home administrators have expressed concern about such competition and the adequacy of care provided in swing-bed hospitals, the empirical evidence currently available shows that such competition exists at most in isolated communities rather than on a widespread basis.

—Geographic access is considerably enhanced by the swing-bed approach in rural areas. In particular, higher proportions of rural residents remain in their home communities after the availability of hospital swing beds than before.

Adequacy of Care

This paper has dealt almost exclusively with the availability dimension of access rather than the adequacy dimension. Nonetheless, some evidence presently exists regarding the adequacy of the swing-bed approach in terms of the quality of long-term care provided.[11] Using quality measures that could range from 0 to 100 percent, the quality of care provided in swing-bed hospitals during the Texas, Iowa, and South Dakota demonstrations was

11. William F. Jessee, "Quality Assurance: Evaluating Services of Small, Swing-Bed Hospitals," *Hospitals*, vol. 56 (November 16, 1982), p. 74; and Peter W. Shaughnessy, Linda D. Breed, and David P. Landes, "Assessing the Quality of Care Provided in Rural Swing-Bed Hospitals," *Quality Review Bulletin*, vol. 8 (May 1982), pp. 12–20.

found to be lower than that provided in comparison nursing homes. The average quality score for nursing homes was 68 percent, compared with 64 percent for swing-bed hospitals. Although the difference was not substantial, it was statistically significant and largely attributable to less adequate treatment of psychosocial problems in swing-bed hospitals. In fact, the treatment of medical and subacute problems was more adequate in swing-bed hospitals than in nursing homes. A larger study comparing patient outcomes between nursing home and swing-bed patients is ongoing.[12]

Urban Swing Beds

Although patterns of and interrelations among demand, use, supply, financing, and regulatory factors are different between rural and urban communities, the strength of the access results presented here points to the potential value of the swing-bed approach in urban areas. First, the tendency of rural swing-bed hospitals to gravitate to a more intense medical case mix than nursing homes suggests that urban hospitals would do the same under a swing-bed program. In fact, urban hospitals would likely gravitate to an even greater level of case-mix intensity because of their service capabilities.

Second, it is apparent that swing beds are widely used as holding beds for long-term care patients in need of some degree of rehabilitation until they can be discharged home, possibly under the care of a home health nurse, or discharged to another long-term care bed if necessary. In view of the willingness and capacity of swing-bed hospitals to treat more intense medical needs, this holding-bed phenomenon might be to the benefit of patients and payers alike. That is, long-term care patients who can be rehabilitated enough to return home after a relatively short stay in an urban swing-bed hospital might never be admitted to a nursing home environment, where health care practices are naturally influenced by treating more patients who stay permanently or for considerable lengths of time.

At a minimum, it appears that experimentation with the swing-bed approach in larger and urban hospitals may be warranted, especially in view of the recent increases in transitional-care beds as a result of hospitals converting acute-care beds to hospital-based SNF beds. It is unclear whether hospital swing beds in urban areas would compete directly with nursing homes or even

12. Shaughnessy and others, *Hospital Swing Beds in the United States.*

home care, although such competition might be beneficial. It would be possible to use different reimbursement methods, including an all-inclusive acute-care and long-term care payment. If an experiment were conducted with selected hospitals in certain locations, it would afford the opportunity to assess whether the quality of combined acute and SNF care is enhanced. In all, owing to the powerful effects of the prospective payment system on both acute and subacute long-term care delivery systems, experimentation with alternative methods of paying for and providing swing-bed care in urban and larger hospitals now appears appropriate.[13] It may well be that a carefully planned demonstration and evaluation program could simultaneously examine the relative costs and benefits of swing-bed care, hospital-based and freestanding SNF care, home care, and different approaches to reimbursing for each in urban areas.

Comments by Raymond Coward

I HAVE put aside all of my concerns about the methodology that was used in the study and have concentrated my remarks on two particular policy issues that the paper raised in my mind. Those two issues were: (1) the comparative ability of swing beds to respond to the long-term care needs of the rural elderly; and (2) the generalizability of swing beds as a policy solution to the problems of long-term care access for the elderly in rural society.

The Continuum of Care

Since the early 1970s, the need for, and advantages of, a "continuum of care" approach to delivering long-term care services has been debated widely. Of course, it has taken much longer to transform this rhetoric into reality and in many places a large majority of the pieces of the continuum are only now emerging and being put into place. Nowhere is this more true than in the small towns and rural communities of the nation, where there continues to be a narrower range of all services available.

What concerns me about much of the "access" debate surrounding swing-bed programs is the narrowness of the comparisons that are being drawn—that is, too frequently the policy comparisons have focused exclusively on nursing homes versus hospital-

13. The possibility of an urban swing-bed demonstration is under active consideration by HCFA, which is, however, awaiting the results of the ongoing evaluation of the rural swing-bed program, as noted in Shaughnessy and others, *Hospital Swing Beds in the United States*.

based swing-bed programs, a comparison of a very narrow range of the full continuum.

For example, as I examine the data presented by Shaughnessy on activities of daily living and instrumental activities of daily living, I am less impressed by the magnitude of the differences between rural elders in swing-bed programs and those in nursing homes. I am more struck by the similarity of disability prevalences that are reported for swing-bed patients and those that I have observed in populations that are being served at home by community-based services. These data clearly indicate that there is a segment of rural elders whose medical needs and degree of severity can benefit from the more intensive services that are available in hospital-based programs. But, as I look at the medical or nursing problems discussed in the Shaughnessy paper, I am taken most by the large numbers of elders in these samples who seem to be operating at a functional "medically intense" level that would make them excellent candidates for home-based services if such services existed in their community.

Shaughnessy states in the beginning of his paper that he is interested in relative access—obviously, however, the critical elements are relative to what and access to what? Whereas 90 percent of swing-bed patients have stays of less than thirty days, only one-third of nursing home patients have stays of this duration. What, then, are the exact services to which access needs improving? Perhaps a better comparison for swing beds is to the short-term, posthospital discharge, community-based alternatives that are being created and implemented in many areas (including small towns and rural communities) in our nation.

Shaughnessy makes the comparison to rural nursing home patients—a relevant and absolutely critical comparison, but not the only comparison with meaning for the policymaker. I am not trying to pit a supposedly perfect community-based system against "institutionalization," a term with sinister connotations. Rather, I am trying to raise the limitations of a narrow comparison in order to arrive at a better understanding of the comparability of different alternatives. In Vermont, the swing-bed option does not get debated and compared only with nursing homes; rather, it is debated in a policy context that is much more diverse. Policymakers are asked to make choices between a range of alternatives, not simply from these two particular options. The debate surrounding access to long-term care for rural elders will be fully comprehended only when comparisons can be drawn among all the major relevant alternatives.

Within this broader comparative context, many of the same issues raised by Shaughnessy will be relevant in the broader policy analysis context—for example, maintaining contact with, and access to, the family support network; the appropriateness of level of care to the needs of elders being served; and competition and segmentation of the market.

Generalizability

The second point about which I wish to raise concerns is the generalizability of the swing-bed option. For the sake of argument, I am prepared to accept the contention that permitting small rural hospitals the option of using their acute-care beds in this manner has economic advantages for the hospitals, provides needed services for some elders, and improves access to some kinds of long-term care for the residents of the communities the hospitals serve.

What I caution against is the contention (which Shaughnessy does not make) that this option is a major answer to the problems of access to long-term care for rural elders. As in all panaceas, this is not the preferred solution for every community. One must seek a policy understanding to determine exactly where this solution is most effectively applied. Obviously, swing beds cannot be the solution to the problems of access for the 100 rural counties in this nation that do not even have a physician, let alone a hospital. Nor can swing beds be the solution for the 338 rural communities whose hospitals closed between 1972 and 1982. And I will argue that swing beds will not provide access to the services that are most needed by the 60 percent of rural elders who are receiving the majority of their long-term care from their families. Thus there are many thousands of rural communities for which swing beds are not a viable option nor the preferred means of solving their access problems.

Moreover, those rural communities where there are no hospital facilities or who have recently lost their community hospital are frequently the most economically disadvantaged and chronically depressed areas. Remember, there is evidence to suggest that many of the rural communities that are able to maintain a hospital already are a cut above most small towns and rural communities. Some of the aged face a quadruple "whammy"—they are old and poor and live in a chronically depressed, rural community. For those, I doubt that swing beds offer much hope of improving access to the services they need.

As with all bandwagons, there is a concern that the enthusiasm and support for this latest phenomenon will detract from a diligent search for still other new and creative strategies for meeting the long-term care needs of rural elders. Public policy must allow for, indeed encourage and provide incentives for, the further exploration of still other innovative alternatives and the creation of a continuum of responses to their access needs.

Comments by James R. Knickman

I WOULD like to make a few suggestions about the data and methods used in the paper. Although some of the comments suggest alternative methodological approaches, I want to emphasize that Shaughnessy's findings, as presented, are valuable and valid. My comments focus on considerations relevant for using the research framework to answer additional questions.

I found the classification that he develops very useful. Dividing variables into case-mix, service-mix, and patient-mix categories allows for an organized and comprehensive look at the swing-bed population. However, it would be useful to know which variables are not significantly different for the two groups of patients in addition to the list of those that are significant. It is just as interesting to know how the patients are similar as how they are different.

It should be noted that the comparison sample of nursing homes could have patient mixes that are not exactly comparable to a randomly selected set of rural nursing homes. This is possible because the comparison nursing homes are all within fifty miles of a swing-bed hospital. The case mix of these nursing homes might be influenced by the fact that there are swing-bed hospitals close by. Some of the patients treated in the swing beds might have been treated in the comparison nursing homes had there been no swing beds. Because of this, I think the comparison group of nursing homes should have been from areas where there were no swing beds close by.

The paper begins with a discussion of hypotheses about access and competition, but I do not think the data set allows good tests of access hypotheses. To study access, it is most appropriate to use population-based data. Two populations, in two distinct areas, one where swing beds are present and one where they are not, are needed in order to definitively test hypotheses about the effects of swing beds on access and utilization rates. If only case-mix variables are considered, as is done in the paper, by definition you are only looking at that part of the population that is comprised of users. This ignores the part of the population that does not use services.

The key access question is what happens to swing-bed type patients when there are no swing beds available? There are four possibilities. They could receive treatment in acute-care hospitals while awaiting placements in nursing homes. They could be treated in the community, as discussed earlier. Third, they could go to nursing homes, competing for space with other patients. Or fourth, they could receive no treatment at all.

An analysis of which of these four outcomes occurs in the absence of swing beds is essential in evaluating the impact of swing beds on access. I hope that in his future research Shaughnessy can do this analysis to complement the useful comparison of patient characteristics presented in this paper.

Let me close with some comments concerning the competition issue. The paper basically concludes that there is not much competition because patients treated in swing beds have a different case mix and a different set of needs than patients treated in nursing homes in the area. Another possibility, however, is that there is no competition only because there is excess demand for long-term care services in these rural areas. If swing beds are opened in areas where there is no excess demand, competition with nursing homes might occur.

Another form of competition to consider might be between expansion of long-term care capacity through swing beds versus expansion through the marginal increase of nursing home beds at existing facilities (such as the construction of a new wing). If beds are added to the margin of existing nursing homes, many of the fixed costs discussed in the Finkler paper can be avoided. The analysis presented in the paper does not allow a test of the hypothesis that swing beds slow the growth of new nursing home beds in rural areas.

In addition, one other type of competition to consider is that between swing-bed care and community-based care. An analysis of the trade-offs between swing beds and either extra beds at existing nursing homes or community-based services would be interesting to explore.

Quality of Care

HELEN L. SMITS

THE QUALITY of the care given in nursing homes has been the subject of national debate for the past fifteen years. A series of shocking and well-publicized scandals in the early 1970s has left an impression, a full fifteen years later, with both the general public and many professionals that nursing homes are "bad" and that aggressive and detailed regulation is the only solution to their universal problem. In this context, the use of swing beds has a great advantage: the care delivered there exists outside of the public myths about nursing homes. Both consumers and professionals can, as a result, view what occurs with unbiased eyes.

Despite the general perception, there is evidence that institutional long-term care in the United States has made great strides over that same fifteen years. Aggressive regulatory efforts by the states and the federal government that began in the early 1970s appear to have markedly decreased the incidence of shocking abuse or neglect. A recent study by the Institute of Medicine affirms the need to continue regulatory efforts, but notes that "although the incidence of neglect and abuse is difficult to quantify, the collective judgment of informed observers, including members of the committee and of resident advocacy organizations, is that these disturbing practices now occur less frequently."[1]

Students, and their academic institutions, have shown a new interest in the field of geriatrics. As a result there are now a number of young physicians and nurses who are both well trained in caring for the elderly and eager to do so. At the same time, there has been a marked improvement in understanding of the medical needs of the elderly and of the functional problems resulting from physical impairment. Finally, and perhaps most important, nursing home residents themselves have begun to say, in no uncertain terms, what they think about the care they receive.

1. Institute of Medicine, Committee on Nursing Home Regulation, *Improving the Quality of Care in Nursing Homes* (Washington, D.C.: National Academy Press, 1986), p. 3.

In order to evaluate the quality of care given in swing beds, one must begin by defining high-quality nursing home care as that term is understood in 1986. I will then review, both from the data and from my personal experience in visiting swing-bed hospitals, what kind of care is being given in some of the small and rural hospitals that now participate in the swing-bed program.

What is quality?

Quality of care in the long-term setting has three essential elements: the quality of the basic medical and nursing services, the quality of functional and rehabilitation assessment efforts, and the quality of life.

Basic Medical and Nursing Services

Residents of nursing homes, whether long stay or short stay, need high-quality medical and nursing care. Perhaps the most important lesson learned from the British geriatricians is that there are no "typical" complaints of the elderly that should be dismissed as unimportant solely because of the patients' age. Dizziness, memory loss, weight loss, and decrease in energy levels, just to name a few, deserve evaluation in the 80-year-old just as they do in the 40-year-old. A careful, critical approach to patient management can define, in many instances, conditions that can be ameliorated or treated.

Of the many elements of geriatrics, one of the most important for institutional care is a careful approach to pharmacology. When full-scale evaluations of elderly patients are undertaken, as they have been in the geriatric evaluation units of the Veterans' Administration system, one of the commonest "conditions" identified is the overuse of drugs.[2] This includes both the use of too many drugs without adequate consideration of their interactions and the use of very standard drugs, such as digitalis, without careful consideration of changed metabolic rates in the elderly.

A full review of geriatric medicine and nursing is an appropriate subject for a textbook and cannot be undertaken here. The central point is simply that the elderly need good physicians and nurses and that care in a nursing home should be at least as good as, if not better than, the care given to ambulatory or hospitalized patients.

---

2. Laurence Z. Rubenstein and others, "Effectiveness of a Geriatric Evaluation Unit: A Randomized Clinical Trial," *New England Journal of Medicine*, vol. 311 (December 27, 1984), pp. 1664–70.

Functional Assessment

A comprehensive assessment of the functional capacity of each resident is an essential element in long-term care. Many methods for undertaking such assessment have been suggested; the most important and well known is the simple scale known as the activities of daily living (ADL), first proposed by Katz over twenty years ago.[3] This assessment must include evaluation of the patient's capacity to function across a variety of dimensions, his or her emotional state, medical conditions and needs, social interactions, and financial situation. This concept is so important that the Institute of Medicine recommended that such assessment become a new regulatory requirement for all institutions.[4]

One of the primary challenges in long-term care arises because no individual professional caregiver has the capacity to conduct the entire assessment; by definition it must be a team effort. Nursing staff have the primary responsibility for conducting assessments, but their evaluation must draw on the physician's history and physical, the social worker's evaluation of finances and available resources, and the physical therapist's evaluation of the patient's capacity to improve motor skills, to name only a few. High-quality care involves not only assessments that have drawn on all necessary professional skills but a recording of those assessments in such a way that all caregivers, including the less skilled, can understand and make use of the information.

Although a good deal of lip service is given to the ADLs, the typical geriatric functional assessment is not common practice among physicians or nurses accustomed to acute care. Although the actual elements are simple, each must be carefully considered; evaluation must be based on a patient and thoughtful period of observation. If, for example, a high premium is placed on having residents dressed by a given time, then the individual who is slow or clumsy may easily be classified as "needing help with dressing" when in fact he or she could manage alone. The same is true of the capacity to feed one's self independently. Evaluation of the instrumental activities of daily living, or those activities needed to function at home, is even more alien to the acute-care nurse. The hospital-based nurse, to put it simply, hardly ever needs to

3. Sidney Katz and others, "Studies of Illness in the Aged: The Index of ADL: A Standardized Measure of Biological and Psychosocial Function," *Journal of the American Medical Association*, vol. 185 (September 21, 1963), pp. 914–19.

4. Institute of Medicine, *Improving the Quality of Care*, p. 77.

think about whether or not a patient could use the telephone at home.

Functional assessment is not difficult or technically complex. It does, however, require some retraining before either nurses or physicians are comfortable with it.

Quality of Life

When residents themselves are asked about what they value in nursing home care, the answers do not focus on the relatively technical aspects of care discussed so far.[5] Instead, areas of importance include staff attitudes, the quality of food, activities, and access to visitors from outside the institution. The ability to make choices—in diet, in when to arise and go to bed, in roommates, and in activities—is clearly essential to any kind of contentment for the long-stay resident.

In 1985 the National Citizens' Coalition for Nursing Home Reform asked able residents to discuss, in a relatively open-ended way, what they valued the most highly in their care and how they thought care in the nation overall might be improved. The resulting document is a rich and fascinating one that should be required reading for all involved in long-term care. The report is full of exactly the kind of comments that you and I would make if we were asked to evaluate a hotel in which we were forced to live over a long period: a cheerful greeting and a hot cup of coffee in the morning are major determinants of satisfaction. Residents are certainly interested in staff's abilities, but that interest tends to focus on the aides and orderlies, those staff to whom the residents are closest. One has a distinct sense that a rich and varied menu, pleasant aides, and interesting activities are of considerably more importance to residents than is the physician who admitted them.

Quality of care in swing beds

The only exhaustive study undertaken of the quality of care in swing beds is that done by Shaughnessy and colleagues in their evaluation of the original swing-bed demonstration.[6] Overall, swing-bed hospitals provided care that was modestly worse than that in a group of nursing homes that had been identified by state

---

5. Joy Spalding, "Analysis of Residents' Discussions: Summary of Findings," in National Citizens' Coalition for Nursing Home Reform, *A Consumer Perspective on Quality Care: The Residents' Point of View* (Washington, D.C.: NCCNHR, 1985).

6. Peter W. Shaughnessy, Linda D. Breed, and David P. Landes, "Assessing the Quality of Care Provided in Rural Swing-Bed Hospitals," *Quality Review Bulletin*, vol. 8 (May 1982), pp. 12–20.

surveyors as providing "average or above average" care. Most of the elements used by the evaluators related to various aspects of technical medical and nursing services. In these areas, the swing-bed hospitals were better than nursing homes at providing services such as laboratory tests and electrocardiograms but were worse than nursing homes in the area of professional nursing and physician care. Perhaps the most important lesson to be learned from this evaluation is that nursing home care, when objectively analyzed, cannot be dismissed as poor in the average institution and that hospital staff have a good deal to learn if they are ever to do a good job in providing long-term care services.

Within this same evaluation, areas relating to functional assessment were studied only within categories described as "physical and occupational therapy" and "sensory compensation." Swing-bed hospitals scored the same as nursing homes on the first and better than nursing homes on the second. In the only measure of the quality of life, "social-recreational," the hospitals did considerably worse than the nursing homes.

In general, this fits both with one's intuitive guess about how hospitals would be likely to perform and with my observations during two visits to groups of swing-bed hospitals in Kansas and Missouri. In the areas of technical medical and nursing care, hospitals have both some natural advantages and some natural disadvantages. The frequent presence of the physician is clearly a great asset, both in terms of the visits required by regulation and in terms of the nursing staff's need to discuss care and discharge planning with the doctor. Greater availability also guarantees prompt evaluation when the patient's condition changes. There is good statistical evidence that many physicians are unwilling to care for nursing home residents; this phenomenon would appear particularly likely to occur in rural settings where nursing homes are often a great distance from a practitioner's base of practice.[7] Swing beds, which are easily accessible to physicians and are located in an institution that is visited frequently, can help to increase continuity of care and the number of physicians willing to continue to care for the institutionalized elderly.

Available physicians are not, however, necessarily good physicians. The physician who cares for both acute- and long-term care patients in the same hospital will need to rethink practice styles and approaches to care for the long-term resident. For

7. David L. Rabin, "Physician Care in Nursing Homes," *Annals of Internal Medicine,* vol. 94 (January 1981), pp. 126–28.

example, the quick drop-in visit every morning, so typical of hospital rounds, is very unlikely to be a satisfactory way to learn about the elderly long-term patient. The same amount of time spent once a week may be much more fruitful. Special attention to training in areas such as the pharmacology of the elderly will also be needed before hospital-based care will reach the level achieved in many nursing homes.

The relatively good scores of swing-bed hospitals on "physical and occupational therapy" in the Shaughnessy evaluation do not convince me that hospital staff are skilled at functional assessments or able to develop care plans based on the results of such assessment. In this area, I suspect that the result of the study can be attributed to the fact that the work was conducted in the mid- to late 1970s and reflects practice standards that have changed since that time. If functional assessment is seen as primarily the responsibility of the rehabilitation departments—that is, as a kind of compart- mentalized event, separate from the rest of care—then hospitals, with active occupational and physical therapists, may well perform better than nursing homes. If, however, functional assessment is viewed, as it should be, as a central element in all of long-term care and one that must be understood and used by all members of the care team, then hospitals are less likely to do well.

My observation on my visits to swing-bed hospitals was that there was a good deal of lip service to "the ADLs" but little real understanding of what they were or how they should be measured. None of the charts I looked at contained a simple, readable ADL form that told me exactly how the patient functioned at the last evaluation and how that function had changed since admission. Such forms are much more common in nursing home charts. Instead, there were likely to be nurses' notes saying "ADLs fine except for dressing," a comment that leaves me with some doubt as to how carefully the other activities have, in fact, been observed.

In addition, hospital nurses were understandably confused about the meaning of the instrumental activities of daily living and how they should be used in evaluating the patient and planning for living arrangements. I saw one unfortunate resident who was in reasonably good health and whose mental state was good except for some absentmindedness. She was destined for a nursing home because she had forgotten a cake she was baking, burned it, and frightened her landlord, who now refused to take her back. A creative discharge planner could come up with a wide range of solutions to that particular problem, including a timer to turn the oven off; the story means in effect that the landlord had made the placement decision, and I doubt that he was much of a judge.

In the area of quality of life, the relatively hectic pace of even a small hospital is clearly a major barrier to good care for the longer-term resident. As anyone who has been a hospital patient knows, there are some mornings when large numbers of admissions or a shortage of nursing staff make the hot cup of coffee and the relaxed and cheerful "good morning" impossible to come by.

The absence of basic recreational facilities was clearly a problem in those institutions studied in the original evaluation as well as in almost all of those institutions that I visited. Problems in planning and executing recreational activities for one or two residents at a time were raised by staff in almost every facility I visited. The one exception was those hospitals that either owned a long-term care facility already or had one located very close by. Clearly the best recreation for long-term residents can be provided only when there is a critical mass of residents to undertake projects, participate in discussion groups, or play bingo.

In rural swing-bed hospitals, one great advantage in quality of life is the ability to keep patients within their own community. Where distances between even small towns are great, as they are in the western states I visited, elderly friends and family may find it impossible to visit someone located in a nursing home a hundred miles from home. When that same individual remains in a local hospital, visiting is much easier and the patient can even continue, if his or her condition permits, to participate in the most important community activities such as church services. This advantage was cited by many who work in the swing-bed program as one of the most important reasons to keep the program going.

Implications for quality assurance

The implications of these observations for traditional quality assurance programs are relatively straightforward. In the area of traditional medicine and nursing, such as drug management and prevention of skin breakdown, hospitals are likely to do reasonably well to begin with and are also capable of improving what they do. Audits and monitoring activities will need to focus on generic problems, such as polypharmacy, rather than on the more traditional diagnosis-based methods. This is not, however, a particularly radical change.

In the area of functional assessment there is still a great deal to be done. I would recommend that every swing-bed institution begin the quality assurance process by identifying and implementing a record-keeping system for functional status. Such a system may be very simple and straightforward: a one- or two-page checklist is sufficient. Use of the checklist need not be based on elaborate training: a process of verifying one another's observations and resolving differences in opinion can do a great deal to ensure that all staff, especially all nursing staff, are competent in conducting such assessments. Experts in functional assessment are not hard to find in swing-bed hospitals since physical and occupational therapists are always available. In addition, swing-bed hospitals would be well advised to take the truly radical step of asking area nursing homes to give them assistance in mastering these techniques, which are standard practice in the long-term care setting.

In the area of quality of life, swing-bed hospitals need to continue to work on the areas in which they are at a natural disadvantage while emphasizing and strengthening those areas in which they naturally do well. Some creative approaches to patient care are often needed. For example, one institution found that the provision of routine care during the early morning hospital rush simply didn't work for the swing-bed patients and therefore shifted such care, including bathing, to evenings, when staff had more available time.[8]

Organized activities will continue to present a serious problem because of the small numbers of residents involved. Hospitals that do not themselves own or operate a long-term care facility would do well to see if they could share activities with area nursing homes. Efforts should also be made to see that patients participate, as much as is possible, in community activities. Sending a patient out of the hospital to church is an alien concept to hospital staff, but is well worth the effort for many long-stay patients.

The quality of life is an essential element in good long-term care; it contributes to the process of recovery and makes return home possible. Although swing-bed residents are, in many instances, "short-stay" residents, these short stays are measured in weeks and months, not a few days. The inconveniences everyone is asked to tolerate in very brief hospital stays are simply not acceptable over the longer term, particularly when the sense of alienation and isolation that result from poor quality of life can contribute directly to poor outcomes.

The question of regulation

A good deal has been made of the relatively modest exemptions from the nursing home conditions of participation made for swing-bed hospitals. Nursing homes, quite understandably, feel discriminated against when competing institutions are not held to

8. William F. Jessee, "Quality Assurance: Evaluating Services of Small, Swing-Bed Hospitals," *Hospitals,* vol. 56 (November 16, 1982), pp. 74–77.

the same standards as they are. In fact, I believe that the real regulatory effect on swing beds comes not from the official release from specific conditions but from the fact that inspectors are much less concerned about the neglect or abuse of patients in hospitals and therefore approach inspection of swing beds with a more positive attitude than is the case in many nursing homes. Most inspectors quite freely admit that they first form an intuitive notion of what is going on in an institution and then seek violations (or the lack of them) to confirm that underlying belief. In addition, inspectors visiting a swing-bed hospital may have the time to review the care records of all of the long-term residents currently present, an arrangement that helps to focus the inspection on the actualities of resident care.

But the current standards are not cast in stone. There has been a growing consensus, over the past few years, that nursing home conditions of participation ought to become more "outcome oriented" or more directly centered on observation or review of the care actually given to residents. The consensus tends to break down as soon as the concept is made more specific, but in fact I believe we can expect with reasonable certainty that a more outcome-oriented set of standards will be in place sometime within the next five years.

The effect of a change in standards on swing beds should be interesting. If a system were developed which evaluated care in the same way that the Shaughnessy group evaluated the demonstrations, then outcome-oriented standards would provide a challenge to swing-bed hospitals to bring their standards of care up to that of "average or above average" nursing homes. While replication of the Shaughnessy work for regulatory purposes seems unlikely, some form of outcome-oriented regulation does not. An outcome-oriented system of inspection would both challenge hospitals to improve the quality of their long-term care and help hospitals to answer a question with which they have been wrestling: exactly what type of patients should be cared for in swing beds? While I do not believe that there is a single simple answer to that question, it is apparent that swing beds, at least as they now operate in small hospitals, cannot expect to provide the full range of services to all residents.

The use of swing beds has taught everyone some interesting lessons. The first, and most surprising to some people, is the fact that nursing home care in this country isn't dreadful; at least a well-selected group of "average to above average" nursing homes appears to give quite good care when studied objectively. The second lesson is that the provision of chronic care is not easy. Put together, those lessons mean that hospitals can learn something from nursing homes. And it is that last lesson, the diminution of the biases that have kept nursing home staff and residents out of the perceived "mainstream" of health care, which is perhaps the most important of all. Put simply, chronic care is not separate from the rest of health care, and all care will benefit from an increased understanding of that fact.

Comments by Catherine Hawes

As OTHER contributors have observed, the task of providing services to the elderly who need long-term care is extremely complex. It is challenging not only in terms of the kinds of care individuals need but also in terms of the pressures providers face. On the one hand, providers must cope with intense pressure to contain costs. On the other, they are expected to deal with an increasingly complex population, one with a mix of acute, subacute, and chronic-care needs. Further, they are expected to provide care that enhances patients' physical, mental, and emotional well-being, as well as their capacity to function as independently as possible despite the presence of diseases or disabilities. Finally, institutional long-term care providers are expected to meet these multiple needs in a safe environment that fosters independence and high quality of life. Thus providing long-term care is not an easy task, whether by a nursing home or hospital.

As Helen Smits notes, acute-care institutions face a particular challenge, since in general they are accustomed to providing time-limited, diagnosis-centered interventions that are largely physician-dominated. This is not the style sought in long-term care, in which a team approach to multidimensional patient needs assessment, care planning, and service provision is the model.

While hospital personnel obviously strive to deliver care in a humane manner, attention to quality of life, multidimensional needs assessment, physical functioning, and other aspects of high-quality long-term care has not been a predominant concern in the acute-care sector. Thus hospitals providing long-term care must revise their concept of quality, as well as modify their quality assurance systems.

Since Smits has elegantly described the essential components of quality in long-term care, I intend to focus on two other basic issues. What do we know about the quality of care provided in swing beds? What are the policy implications of these findings?

In her paper, Smits describes a prior evaluation of the HCFA demonstrations by the University of Colorado Center for Health Services Research and her own impressions based on site visits to some of the Robert Wood Johnson Foundation grantee hospitals. I concur with much of what she argues about the strengths and weaknesses of hospital swing-bed performance relative to high-quality long-term care. I would argue, however, that the important comparison is not so much between the performance of hospital swing beds and nursing homes as it is between what all long-term care providers "ought" to be doing for patients and what they are doing.

Now, what are the policy implications of Smits's paper? The first policy assertion I would make is that regulation is essential. It is not particularly popular, and is perhaps even anachronistic, to say that in these times, but regulation is necessary for a variety of reasons. One of the most important roles of regulation is to clarify the concept of what high-quality (or acceptable quality) long-term care is—whether it is provided in hospital swing beds or in nursing homes. Providing appropriate, high-quality, long-term care is very different from much of what hospitals traditionally do. Thus, as prior research and observation suggest, hospitals need guidelines, particularly in areas such as psychosocial care, activities, quality of life, multidimensional needs assessment, and care planning. So I think it is important to have explicit regulations that address these issues and set clear performance standards for providers.

My second policy conclusion is that current certification standards for medicare and medicaid are inadequate to this task. Each of the two hospitals I visited met current resource input standards, but their organization, orientation, patient mix, and daily practices led to significantly different patterns of care, different areas of satisfactory or outstanding performance, and different areas of needed improvement. Current federal standards should be expanded to include individual patient needs assessment and care planning, quality of life issues, and residents' rights. This latter, in particular, is a foreign concept in many hospitals.

My third conclusion is that we need to move much more toward process and outcome standards. Revising current regulations so that they specify appropriate process care standards and define desirable and achievable patient outcomes is likely to be much more useful in educating swing-bed providers and improving quality of care.

Fourth, I suggest that while Joint Commission on the Accreditation of Hospitals standards and surveys may be useful to hospitals, the swing-bed hospitals, like other long-term care providers and nursing homes, ought to be inspected by state and federal regulatory agencies. This is important both because there are differences in quality standards and also because survey reports should be public information.

Fifth, the survey process should also focus more explicitly on the care patients actually receive, rather than on the capacity of institutions to provide appropriate care. In surveys appropriate process and outcome measures are needed as key indicators of the quality of care an institution provides.

There are two other issues related to regulation that I want to address. The first is whether swing beds ought to be held to the same set of standards as nursing homes. I have mixed feelings about this issue because the answer depends in part on the kinds of patients these institutions serve and their length of stay. Current nursing home standards are widely acknowledged to be minimums, so one is reluctant to suggest that some facilities be exempted. Further, one is reluctant to suggest that certain patients should receive different care—less space or fewer activities, for example. But in general, the fairly minor role of hospitals (in terms of total nursing home bed days) and the typical length of stay of swing-bed patients suggest this is not critical, and I concur with Smits's assessment of this issue. The second issue is whether other hospitals, larger ones or ones not in rural areas, ought to be allowed to participate in the swing-bed program. I do not see this as an issue from the perspective of quality of care. After all, there are large urban nursing homes. Some do terrific jobs, and some do terrible jobs. There is a niggling feeling that an institution's size will have an impact on quality, and indeed it may. But it is not clear from empirical evidence what that effect is. Thus there is no clear reason to expect that larger hospitals would do a worse job of providing long-term care in swing beds.

Let me conclude with two points. First, I think there are other benefits from swing-bed programs. If hospitals learn to provide high-quality care in swing beds, it is likely to have beneficial effects on the care provided to all elderly patients—and maybe even those who aren't elderly. All hospital patients, for example, would benefit from increasing attention to quality of life and psychosocial needs.

The last point relates to the debate about where swing beds fit in the continuum of care. Part of the problem of assessing the quality of care in swing beds relates to how one defines the role of swing-bed hospitals. Are they to be an institution providing highly technical, short-term skilled care to persons discharged from acute-care beds "quicker and sicker"? Or are they to be more like traditional nursing homes—serving both short- and long-stay patients, providing access where appropriate care is unavailable and offering a potential solution to bed shortages? Unfortunately, this issue is not being directly addressed. The issues of swing-bed costs and reimbursement seem more pressing than their potential for filling a significant gap in the long-term care continuum.

Perhaps the debate about the role of hospitals and expansion of the swing-bed program can contribute to a genuine debate about action to correct the fragmentation and rigidity of the current long-term care "nonsystem." As a nation, we have devoted an enormous amount of ingenuity and time to a giant shell game, in which long-term care costs of the elderly are shifted from one payer to another and from one institution to another. Definitions of eligibility for services, levels of care, and institutional roles have more to do with financing—who will pay and, more important, who won't—than with the needs of the elderly. For policymakers who are genuinely concerned about quality of care, the fundamental issue is how to redesign the entire system to be patient-centered, so that programs and institutions are more flexible and responsive to the actual care needs of older persons who are sick and often frail.

Swing beds can be an important component of a realistic, appropriate system for providing long-term care that meets the multidimensional needs of the elderly and disabled. But if policy-makers merely want one other way station that the elderly can be shifted from or to in this shell game of who will pay, it will not improve quality or enhance the well-being of individuals who need long-term care.

Comments by Jacqueline Ann John

HEALTH CARE providers have a tendency to focus on the technical aspects of quality. The residents' definition of quality takes for granted the technical aspects and focuses more closely on their individual perception of quality in relation to their own value system.

I believe that the increased interest in gerontology will enhance the quality of care delivered to the geriatric patient in all health care settings. An improved understanding of how the geriatric patient reacts to illness is essential. I am concerned that the criteria adopted to screen appropriateness of services do not reflect a basic understanding of the aging process and frequently restricts access to needed services.

Helen Smits expressed concern about the lack of appropriate functional assessment in the swing-bed program. Kansas and Missouri swing-bed hospitals have worked together to develop and pilot test an assessment tool. Gathering information to facilitate problem identification relating to medical problems, psychosocial needs, and functional limitations is essential in developing an appropriate plan of care for the residents' stay in the facility and an appropriate discharge plan. The care planning process used in the swing-bed program requires establishing measurable goals and an ongoing process of evaluation of patient progress. Short lengths of stay in the swing-bed program, however, do not allow an adequate time frame to monitor long-term changes in functional capability traditionally seen in long-term care institutions.

Many acute-care facilities have upgraded their discharge-planning programs due to the changing incentives created by the medicare prospective payment system and the peer review organizations. Discharge plans must recognize functional impairments if they are to be successful in preventing unnecessary hospital readmissions.

Quality of life is an important consideration in choosing the appropriate placement for residents. Some individuals may benefit by transfer to a facility with more emphasis on functional rehabilitation even though it is away from their home community and may limit family contact. However, the majority of the residents in the swing-bed program prefer to remain close to their family and continue to have the support of their current social structure. For those, that opportunity represents quality of life.

It is true nursing homes can more easily provide group recreational activities because of the number of residents in their facility. Those activities are important because they facilitate the resocialization of those residents into a long-term institutional living arrangement.

Swing-bed residents differ in one important aspect. They are required to enter the program through an episode of illness that results in a three-day acute-care stay. That places those residents at a different point of readiness for recreational programs. They are more receptive to programs that emphasize rehabilitation.

As one compares the swing-bed program with other long-term care institutional programs, one must remember that the missions of the programs differ. The swing-bed program is a transitional program that is meant to bridge between acute care and appropriate postdischarge care. The swing-bed program can best be characterized as extended care. It is not intended to provide a permanent placement option, and in the majority of cases it is not used in that manner.

The swing-bed program is an excellent program for communities that have a shortage of long-term care beds and an excess of hospital beds, especially in those communities that do not have skilled-care beds. Hospitals have the professional expertise and the processes to implement the program. Hospitals willing to provide the administrative and educational support can develop a swing-bed program that will deliver quality care to their residents.

The Meaning of the Swing-Bed Experience

BRUCE C. VLADECK

THE apparent success of swing-bed programs in small rural hospitals, first under the auspices of a Health Care Financing Administration demonstration, then as a matter of statutory policy bolstered by programmatic assistance from the Robert Wood Johnson Foundation, contains a number of significant lessons for the future role and behavior of American hospitals and for public policy toward hospitals. Understood correctly, the swing-bed experience is not an isolated instance of particularistic and specific policies working under particularistic and specific circumstances; instead, it is, or should be, a kind of paradigm for the future evolution of the hospital. The experience with swing beds tells a lot about how hospitals can perform when appropriate standards and expectations for performance, and concomitantly appropriate rewards, are established. The swing-bed experience should provide the basis for a thoroughgoing reassessment of the kinds of roles hospitals should play in the health care system of the future.

As inpatient, acute hospital care has become technologically more sophisticated and more expensive per unit of output, there has been, consciously or not, a narrowing of the conception of what a general hospital can appropriately do. Over time, the perceived jurisdiction of general hospitals has gradually excluded most convalescent care, most physical rehabilitation, most custodial care, and increasingly a larger and larger share of elective surgery and diagnostic procedures. Yet the increasingly narrowly focused general hospital speaks less and less well to the health care needs of a population that is on the whole progressively ever more healthy, yet contains a growing number of persons, many of them elderly, in need of chronic care, convalescent services, and low-intensity rehabilitation.

At the same time, this society as a whole, and thousands of communities within it, has invested countless capital, not only in dollars but in time, energy, and emotional commitment, in the development and maintenance of institutions that the policy savants increasingly conclude are obsolete. The nation, and its

120

communities, is supposed to somehow accept with equanimity the disappearance of a third to half of its hospital stock, just as public policymakers have accepted with apparent equanimity the disappearance of a similar proportion of the national stock of steel-making or textile capacity. At the same time, convertible debentures and industrial revenue bonds are being sold to build new "alternative" health care facilities.

In contrast to these trends, swing beds constitute a small and admittedly fragile reed on which to begin constructing an alternative notion of the hospital, and policy toward hospitals, that is more sensible, more economical, and quite possibly more humane. Such a notion should not ignore the extent to which hospitals have in the past often been ineffective, obtuse, or even incompetent in doing some things, nor the extent to which they have been unnecessarily expensive in doing almost everything. But it should also not ignore the extent to which hospitals as social institutions can be shaped and reshaped to meet social needs as conceptions of those needs change.

The swing-bed experience contains, I would contend, three basic lessons and the germ of one fundamental principle. The three lessons can be simply stated and set aside for awhile for the purposes of discussion, while the fundamental principle is defined, explored, and analyzed. Policy prescriptions then flow from a reintegration of that principle with the prior lessons.

The lessons of swing beds

The first, and entirely nontrivial, lesson of the swing-bed experience is that with appropriate preparation and guidance, and under appropriate professional leadership and regulatory scrutiny, even relatively small and resource-poor hospitals can learn to do, reasonably well, things they had not done before or at least not done recently. Extended care of geriatric patients is, as the early developers of swing beds quickly learned, a fundamentally different service from acute medical-surgical care, and HCFA and the Robert Wood Johnson Foundation have been quite correct, since their earliest involvement with swing beds, in insisting that hospitals recognize those differences and learn how to provide extended care. But, with appropriate carrots, including support for staff training and administrator education as well as reimbursement incentives, and sticks, in terms of certification requirements and survey procedures, hospitals appear to have done so.[1] That is not a small matter.

1. Peter W. Shaughnessy and others, *Hospital Swing Beds in the United States: Initial Findings* (Denver: University of Colorado Center for Health Services Research, November 1985).

Many institutions are incapable of doing more than one thing, or at least of doing more than one thing well (and one hastens to suggest that some institutions, like prisons or high schools, may not be able to do anything well most of the time). Health care professionals and policymakers, especially those with experience within hospitals, have often been highly skeptical about hospitals' capacity to provide services other than those with which they are most familiar. The experience with hospital ventures into organized ambulatory care or community psychiatry, to take just two examples, has not, on balance, been particularly encouraging in this regard. But the evidence with swing beds does seem to be more positive.

Second, perhaps unsurprisingly, the experience of swing beds appears to demonstrate that, under the appropriate circumstances, sunk capital is cheaper than new, and fixed overhead costs can be spread more broadly than they generally are. Services added at the margin, in other words, may incur only marginal costs, all other things being more or less equal.[2] With a hospital industry now operating well below optimal productive capacity, and with continued pressures to constrain costs most acutely felt precisely in those public programs with the greatest expected increase in demand, that is not a trivial lesson either. Of course, irrational pricing policies, interpayer conflicts, or particular circumstances may create situations, possibly quite numerous, in which marginal service increments create much greater than marginal costs, but that will not always be the case.

Third, the experience of swing beds, as a political and policy phenomenon at least as much as a clinical one, should again remind jaded urbanites and suburbanites that important values, quite possibly including therapeutic ones, are promoted by arrangements that make it possible for people to receive services relatively close to home, especially when they *feel* at home. As the problems of the health care system increasingly come to be dominated by the "soft" psychosocial and emotional needs of the chronically ill and their caregivers (as opposed to the clinically and technologically "harder" and more discrete interventions of the tertiary-care hospital), there will be an increased need to find ways to make "at-homeness" an explicit variable in service design and to provide substitutes for a sense of community and mutual caring when the real thing is not available. Receiving care close to home facilitates not only visiting but participation in the care

2. Peter W. Shaughnessy and others, *An Evaluation of Swing Bed Experiments to Provide Long-Term Care in Rural Hospitals*, vol. 1 (Denver: University of Colorado Center for Health Services Research, March 1980).

process itself by family and friends, minimizes the dislocating effects of institutionalization, and increases the probability of maintaining a real continuum of community-based care.

Of course, it is precisely in the "softer" services that hospitals perform comparatively less well, although in recent years they have been encouraged and rewarded only on the "high-tech" side. There is no logical reason why hospitals cannot do better on these dimensions for all their patients, and the combined pressures of increased competition for patients and growing geriatric case loads may be pushing hospitals in that direction anyway. The swing-bed experience appears to contain the commonsensical lesson that it is not hard to keep the services close to home—and the providers of those services still in business—if doing so is acknowledged as an explicit policy objective, even one that is highly constrained by considerations of cost.

The fundamental principle

These three lessons are important not only for themselves, but for their implications in the context of what was described above as the fundamental principle underlying the swing-bed experience. That principle can be expressed in a number of ways and needs to be defined from a number of perspectives. But put succinctly, it is this: the health care community needs to design (and redesign) its service systems, and the institutions within them, around the needs of the clients they serve, not devote all its energies to matching clients with various needs to a set of rigidly defined institutions. Or, still more succinctly, institutions should fit the needs of the people they are supposed to serve, not the other way around. Institutional configurations should follow patient needs. That apparently truistic statement is, in the context of current policy toward hospitals, nursing homes, and other health care institutions, practically revolutionary.

In their remarkable and moving account of the deinstitutionalization of profoundly handicapped residents of New York's Willowbrook State School, David Rothman and Sheila Rothman recount debates in the professional community that impeded development of community residences for the retarded. Once enforcement of a court order mooted some of those debates by requiring the creation of community-based facilities, specifics of design and program turned out to be relatively less important than the commitment to do *something*. According to the Rothmans:

> In examining the performance of group homes, much of the professional literature continues to think about suitability of placement in terms of characteristics of individual clients. Those returned to an institution from the community were ostensibly too aggressive or

too dependent. But this formulation is analogous to blaming the worker in a factory for an accident or an illness when the lighting is poor or the ventilation inadequate. The point is to design a healthful and safe workplace—and by the same token, to design suitable community programs.

The experience of the Willowbrook class not only demonstrates the feasibility of placing even the most handicapped persons in the community . . . but also illustrates some of the models that might be followed—and in this way helps us to stop thinking about the client and begin thinking about the setting as the determinative element in placement outcomes. The question is not whether the client has one or another disability but whether the group home adopts a consistent and useful model, either one described here or another of equal efficacy. . . . If one design does not work, do not fault the client but alter the environment. However self-evident this may sound, it has to date been anything but received truth in the field.[3]

The issues in posthospital care for the elderly and disabled are somewhat different, but the central point is the same. Services should be designed to meet the needs of clients, rather than blaming or punishing the clients for their failure to fit perfectly into bureaucratically or professionally designed service categories.

An 80-year-old woman who fractures a hip or a 75-year-old man who experiences an uncomplicated myocardial infarction is likely to need four to six weeks of supervised, inpatient therapeutic, convalescent, and rehabilitative services before returning home at whatever maximum functional level is attainable. Yet under current circumstances, in most communities, those patients must spend that period in two or three separate facilities, under the day-to-day management of two or three separate sets of caregivers, because of preconceptions about costs, institutional jurisdiction, and bureaucratic requirements. While these hypothetical patients may pass through a number of clinically distinct stages in the course of their illnesses, there is no particularly strong match between those stages and the prevailing bureaucratic definitions of "appropriate" placement or care.[4] In addition to the very real economic and human costs incurred by the bouncing of patients from one setting to another, such a phenomenon makes sense only if one takes as given some of the less rational characteristics of current patterns of health services organization and finance.

3. David J. Rothman and Sheila M. Rothman, *The Willowbrook Wars* (Harper and Row, 1984), pp. 251–52.
4. Bruce C. Vladeck, *Unloving Care: The Nursing Home Tragedy* (Basic Books, 1980), pp. 134–46.

The ultimate expression of policy pathology in geriatric care is the phenomenon of "alternate-care status," or "alternate levels of care," which is often brought to public attention in terms of the perceived problem of hospital "backlog." Alternate-care patients are those who have been defined, in order to meet the bureaucratic needs of financing programs, to no longer belong in acute-care hospitals, but who cannot be placed, in a timely way, in facilities that are defined as "appropriate." As a general rule, such patients receive only minimal nursing and hotel services, not anything like the services for which they have been determined to have legitimate need, yet the actual costs—as opposed to prices paid—to the health care system are not consequentially different from those that the exact same patients in the exact same beds would incur if they were receiving clinically appropriate care. Only in hospitals with functioning swing-bed programs do they receive those services.

Before the advent of the prospective payment system (PPS), it was variously estimated that somewhere between 3 and 7 percent of all medicare inpatient days involved patients on alternate-care status; the problem is a very large one. The PPS has largely defined such patients out of existence for medicare purposes, although they continue to be a major concern and source of expense for many medicaid programs. Thus estimates of the numbers are harder to come by. There is no reason, however, to believe that the actual "problem" has gotten any smaller.

Levels of care   If one accepts, at least intuitively, the basic notion that institutional services should be organized around the needs of patients who find themselves occupying beds in institutions, as swing-bed programs often appear uniquely to do, the question must then be raised as to why hospitals are not now organized in that way. The answer is twofold, involving both the institutional imperatives that have governed hospital development over the last couple of generations and, far more important, the needs and predilections of the major providers of financing for hospital care.

For at least a generation, general hospitals, responding to the combined impetuses of technological development, physician preference, and reimbursement policies, have been adding capacity in specialized, technologically intensive units while gradually diminishing their capacity to care for nonacute patients. The convalescent and rehabilitation wards found in many hospitals three decades ago were replaced by intensive-care units. Dramatic reductions in tuberculosis and polio altered the patient base. Increasingly sophisticated therapeutic technologies were sought after by attending physicians. Services for the chronically ill customarily had few advocates within hospitals' power structure.

Most important was the attitude of the payers. The insane and chronically infirm were literal and figurative wards of the state before there was very much health insurance in the United States; from their inception, Blue Cross and other private insurance plans took pains to avoid paying those costs by excluding a variety of chronic conditions, as well as by limiting days of coverage. Medicare benefits were, of course, quite self-consciously modeled on prevailing Blue Cross policies of the 1950s.

Medicaid, and its predecessor Kerr-Mills, posed somewhat more complicated problems. The framers of those policies sought to provide health insurance-type coverage to cash assistance recipients who had historically been primarily the responsibility of state and local governments, but they recognized that, especially insofar as the chronically ill were concerned, the line between medical care and indoor relief—the poorhouse—was exceedingly thin and potentially quite flexible. The psychiatric case was relatively easy to control; medicaid just wouldn't pay for services in a mental institution for persons between the ages of 21 and 65. But long-term care was much tougher.

At first, medicaid sought to limit its benefits to those that appeared to be medical by covering only "skilled" nursing homes. Without an established professional consensus as to just what that meant, and under considerable pressure from sophisticated state officials, Congress in 1965 left a hole big enough to drive several trucks through. Simultaneously, a liberal interpretation of "skilled" nursing care by the first generation of medicare administrators encompassed a large proportion of all then-existing nursing homes, leaving medicaid to cover the whole lot. Attempting to rationalize this situation, in 1967 Congress invented the category of "intermediate care," but placed the benefit not in title XIX, but in the catch-all title XI of the Social Security Act; only in 1972 was the coverage of intermediate-care facilities incorporated into medicaid.[5]

The point of this history is that none of the levels of care in chronic geriatric services about which policymakers talk so freely, and to which they devote so much energy in defining and enforcing, has very much basis in either clinical realities or empirical experience. The major motivation behind the original classification of levels of care for medicare and medicaid, which

5. Ibid.

now sometimes appears to health care professionals as some sort of holy writ, was the desire by officials at various levels of government to let the other guys pay.

There is now an entire subindustry of peer review organization staff, utilization review coordinators, discharge planners, claims reviewers, software salesmen, and consultants organized around the pseudoscience of assigning patients to levels of care. The driving force behind the entire enterprise is the desire on the part of payers to avoid paying for parts of the care rendered during episodes of illness, and the desire on the part of health care providers to minimize the number of cases for which they are not fully paid. As an unavoidable historical digression, it was as part of this enterprise that diagnosis-related groups (DRGs) were born.

The advent of medicare's prospective payment system has, of course, changed all the rules. For a decade, the issue of levels of care was largely a charade: hospitals, operating under cost-based medicare reimbursement to begin with, received the same payment for most alternate-care days that they received for acute-care days, while professional standards review organizations could certify alternate-care status with the same avidity that American officers counted Vietnamese bodies and could claim that their efforts would be winning the war against medicare costs if only state officials were not so obstructionist as to prevent the further proliferation of nursing home beds. Now, so long as alternate-care status occurs within length-of-stay trim points for the DRGs, medicare is indifferent, in narrow financial terms. It also appears to be indifferent in broader programmatic and human terms as well. Of course, since there are no good DRGs for rehabilitation services, defining those levels of care will be the next focus of attention in response to the eagerness with which hospitals will leap through that loophole.

A continuum of care?

In contrast to the current state of affairs, one could depict, of course solely for purposes of exercising the imagination, what patient-centered long-term geriatric services might look like. To begin with, it is impossible to avoid the buzzword of "continuity." While many different caregivers, at one or several sites, may necessarily be involved with any given case, the patient is much better served and care is delivered more effectively and efficiently when those caregivers share common information, care plans, and objectives. Often, continuity is best ensured when a single professional—be it (too rarely) a personal physician, a discharge coordinator, or a "case manager"—supervises the case over an extended period of time, but such a formal mechanism may not always be necessary. What is crucial is that the individual patient not become a sort of pinball, bouncing back and forth among different institutions with differing objectives and orientations.

Patient-centered services for older people needing long-term care must also be flexible, responsive, and adaptable. The condition of frail, elderly people tends to be highly unstable and highly vulnerable to external shocks of a variety of kinds; what works clinically one day may be entirely inappropriate the next as the patient's needs change. Nor is such change predictably unidirectional; the simplistic notion of a "continuum of care" as a kind of ladder down which patients predictably progress, while appropriate to some cases, runs counter to the limited evidence about the natural history of disability among the elderly. There is a considerable flow of patients not only from hospitals to nursing homes but also from nursing homes to hospitals.

The inherent instability in the condition of many of the frail elderly is exacerbated, of course, by discontinuities and rigidities in the system of caring for them. For chronically ill people living in the community or in nursing homes, for instance, the shock and dislocation of hospitalization in and of itself may have more deleterious long-term consequences than the acute illness that engenders the hospitalization. "Transfer trauma" is a well-documented, if avoidable, problem in many institutional admissions.

In principle, effective swing-bed programs should minimize, or at least mitigate, these problems. The very fact that the patient remains in the same institution over two or more "levels" of care is itself a consequential advantage; when the maintenance of the patient in the same institution also entails continuity in case management, if only by maintaining the interest and involvement of the attending physician, so much the better.

As managers of swing-bed programs know, not all elderly patients preparing to leave "acute" status are likely to benefit from short-stay extended care, and some patients in need of institutional care are indeed moving regularly along a continuum of uninterrupted functional decline. There is an appropriate patient base for long-stay, low-intensity residential institutions providing a kind of service inappropriate to swing beds in a general hospital setting. But just as not all geriatric patients in need of postacute services are good candidates for swing beds, so most such patients are not really good candidates for long-term nursing home placement, and the availability of swing beds for this latter group adds considerable continuity and flexibility to their care.[6]

Another desirable attribute of long-term geriatric services, which may be harder to attain in swing-bed programs, though not impossible, is a much greater degree of real interdisciplinary and interprofessional collaboration than generally prevails in the acute-care hospital setting, in freestanding nursing homes, or in most home care cases. The frail elderly typically have multiple, interactive problems involving not only medical conditions narrowly defined, but also functional, psychological, social, and emotional concerns. Swing-bed units in general hospitals offer a greater potential for coordinated, multiple involvement by nurses, social workers, therapists, and aides than other long-term care settings because the other professionals are literally *there* more often. Physicians who never set foot in nursing homes may go to the hospital every day. On the other hand, physician-dominated decisionmaking of the kind that generally prevails in hospitals is often inappropriate in long-term care, so swing-bed managers face an enormous task of education and diplomacy in realizing the potential for interdisciplinary teamwork that exists in a swing-bed setting.

Of course, the failure of the health care system to provide adequate continuity, flexibility, and teamwork in care of the elderly is not solely a consequence of institutional narrowness or inertia, professional turf guarding, or even individual obtuseness. Financing has a lot to do with it. If one is clever, lucky, and working in the right political subdivision, it is now occasionally possible to piece together adequate financing for continuous, comprehensive, high-quality long-term geriatric services. At a minimum, doing so takes a lot of time and energy that might more productively be devoted to taking care of people. In many communities, arranging adequate financing is simply impossible, no matter how energetic and clever one is.

Whether integrated financing systems are needed first in order to develop integrated long-term care programs, or the programs are needed first in order to figure out the financing arrangements, is one of those chicken-and-egg dilemmas that all too easily becomes an excuse for policy paralysis. But surely the data from

6. Andrew M. Kramer, Peter W. Shaughnessy, and Mary L. Pettigrew, "Cost-Effectiveness Implications Based on a Comparison of Nursing Home and Home Health Case Mix," *Health Services Research*, vol. 20 (October 1985), pp. 387–405.

the swing-bed experience contain ample evidence of the possibility of integrating different financing sources in support of integrated-care programs, while suggesting that such integration may actually, in the aggregate, save money.[7] The problem, of course, continues to be the political unwillingness of A (read medicare or medicaid) to spend one dollar to save two of B's (read medicaid or medicare). In that stalemate, the elderly, especially the poor elderly, are held hostage.

Learning from swing beds

The people who run America's hospitals—administrators, trustees, officials of the increasingly elaborate corporate superstructures in the burgeoning multi-institutional systems—are confused and anxious about the future of their institutions. Demand for acute inpatient services, the basic stock in trade, has been falling precipitously, with no bottom apparently in sight. Consultants and salesmen talk confidently of the closure of one quarter to one half of all hospitals within the next couple of decades. Traditional sources of capital are threatened by tax reform legislation and changes in reimbursement policy, while the imperatives of technological advance, with its frequent concomitant appetite for new capital, appear to be, if anything, accelerating. An increasing supply of physicians contains a goodly number who appear eager to compete with the hospital for revenues, while a new generation of health maintenance organizations, third-party entrepreneurs, and mobilized purchasers of group insurance appear set on prospering by taking business away from the hospitals.

Policymakers appear, from the hospitals' perspective, indifferent, or worse. After at least a generation of excessive openhandedness toward hospitals, they appear, perhaps predictably, to be overreacting in the opposite direction. As short-term budgetary pressures drive all other concerns out of the policy process, the often-stated recognition that outpatient and chronic care services need to be expanded while the acute inpatient sector is shrunk becomes increasingly hollow. Persons in need of services for which a need for expansion is generally recognized fall through the holes in the safety net.

The general public, so far as anyone can tell, shares policymakers' concerns with rising costs and prices and shows an increasing willingness to alter long-established patterns of care, while remaining supportive not only of hospitals in general and of "their" hospital in "their" town, but also of measures to ensure

7. Shaughnessy and others, *An Evaluation of Swing Bed Experiments.*

the availability of hospital services to others. Charitable giving, both in cash and in volunteer services, appears to be at an all-time high, while voters in a number of communities have shown a perhaps surprising willingness to tax themselves additionally to support public hospital services.

In this context, swing beds, while a limited concept of finite potential, appear to hold great promise, both in themselves and as examples of the broader lessons and principles enumerated earlier. Matching, as they do, underutilized but plentiful resources with unmet needs, often at marginal cost below average cost in other kinds of settings, swing beds have made available services to people who might otherwise not have gotten them, or at least not have gotten them in a comparably desirable way.

Should the swing-bed model be extended to larger hospitals? To urban hospitals? To services other than those within the current scope of the medicare skilled nursing facility benefit? Of course. But in a sense those are the wrong questions, embodying and reinforcing the implicit logic of institutional rigidity and levels of care that the swing-bed experience appears to be disproving. Should all hospitals in all communities operate swing-bed programs? Of course not. Only those that can do a good job, in communities where no one is doing the job better. Does the apparent success of swing beds mean that nursing homes as institutions are obsolete? No: the evidence is clear that swing beds and nursing homes serve fundamentally different populations. Does growth of swing beds remove the pressure to build new nursing homes? Perhaps, but new nursing homes are not being built in any event, regardless of growing demand.

Even if the medicare law were amended to permit swing beds in all hospitals, and even if every state enacted appropriate additional implementing legislation, however, adequate financing for swing-bed services would still not be generally available. That is a commentary, though, on financing systems, not on the concept of swing beds. So long as policymakers remain concerned solely with enforcing increasingly narrow definitions of what they will pay for, financing any desirable new service will be difficult. On the other hand, it will be interesting to see how quickly prepaid plans move to invent services that look, in all salient characteristics, much like swing beds, if they do in fact begin to enroll any considerable number of patients at high risk for long-term care.

A more serious, longer-term question about the future of swing beds, both in themselves and as a paradigm for other services for the mentally ill, the younger disabled, substance abusers, the socially displaced, and other growing needy populations, is the capacity of people who work in swing-bed programs to continue to develop, refine, and implement more effective and more satisfying ways to care for their patients. It would be Pollyannism to suggest that in the long run those programs that best provide services to people are most likely to survive the exigencies of institutional competition, policy confusion, and financial uncertainty, but there is some underlying rationality to the notion. The converse is more clearly true: if swing-bed programs cannot continue consistently to demonstrate high-quality appropriate services to appropriately selected patients, the concept will not survive, no matter what happens in the institutional, policy, or financing arenas. As has been noted repeatedly since the earliest discussions of swing beds, economic and medical effectiveness is more easily assured than the nontechnological components of quality. The major uncompleted tasks for proponents of swing beds—as, indeed, for the proponents of most long-term care services—are in the area of quality, especially its "softer" dimensions.

Concluding this discussion in terms of human and clinical effectiveness does more than provide a comfortably hedged and ambivalent approach to prognostication in an increasingly unpredictable environment. It also returns to first principles: developing, managing, and somehow figuring out how to pay for services that respond to and accommodate the needs of patients and potential patients, rather than continuing to squeeze round patients into square bureaucratic boxes. To the extent that the experience with swing beds in rural hospitals has taught any lessons about patient-centered services, it has served a vital purpose, the significance of which will endure whether or not swing beds do.

Comments by Stephen Press

THREE years ago, as medicaid director for the state of Connecticut, I participated in a Robert Wood Johnson Foundation project aimed at designing new directions for the medicaid program. During that project I had the opportunity to review and then reject the hospital swing-bed concept as a demonstration project for my own state. All the medicaid directors within the group were in agreement, believing that hospital swing beds would lead to higher long-term care costs for their states. Clearly, as data of the Health Care Financing Administration have shown, long-term care provided in hospital-based facilities is twice as costly as that provided in freestanding facilities under the medicare program. As vice-president of the American Health Care Association, I am no longer burdened by any bureaucratic role. My views on swing beds have therefore obviously broadened, but that still hasn't helped me to accept the underlying premise of Bruce Vladeck's paper—that swing beds offer the promise of a great new future for the long-term care patient.

In reviewing his paper, I focused on what he described as the fundamental principle of the swing-bed experience—that health services should be designed to meet the needs of clients. I likewise examined what he identified as the three lessons of swing beds, which I would summarize as (1) that hospitals can learn to carry out extended care; (2) that they are not that costly (although it is difficult to find what they are being compared to); and (3) that swing beds provide positive care for the patient.

I readily accept the principle that health services should be designed to meet the needs of patients and patients should not be forced into the cubbyholes of the health care system. However, Vladeck has not convinced me that this principle is what his paper is all about. I think it is about helping hospitals by sticking long-term care patients in their vacant beds.

I am likewise concerned by his three lessons of swing beds. I certainly cannot quarrel with the premise that hospitals can learn to do things reasonably well that they have not done before. In that context, I am certain that hospitals can and do provide adequate, quality long-term care services. They clearly do so in distinct-part facilities. I would also agree that swing beds may be necessary in some states or localities in the absence of an adequate supply of long-term care beds. Certainly swing beds are better than a total absence of long-term care. I do not disagree that hospitals should have a role in long-term care, but I would have liked to see him describe what that role should be. We at the American Health Care Association are open to discussing the issue and have tried to bridge the gap between hospitals and nursing homes in recent joint meetings, but obviously vast differences remain.

My disagreement begins to arise with Vladeck's second and third lessons: he fails to compare adequately the relative capabilities of swing beds and long-term care facilities in terms of the cost and quality of care in treating long-term care patients.

The paper glosses over the cost issue. "Sunk capital is cheaper than new, and fixed overhead costs can be spread more broadly than they generally are. Services added at the margin, in other words, may incur only marginal costs, all other things being more or less equal." What does all this mean, and are things equal? Does this mean swing beds where there is or can be an adequate supply of long-term beds, and are those swing beds providing comparable services? Does this mean using hospital beds as they are, without expending additional capital to enable hospitals to provide the kind of quality of life nursing homes can provide, such as common dining and recreational facilities? If this means hospitals meeting nursing home standards, one has to look at the costs that hospitals have incurred in renovating older facilities to convert them to long-term care distinct parts. Hospitals that fail to rehabilitate their facilities just can't meet the social and recreational needs of long-term care patients. The point here is that services added at the margin may be insufficient to meet patients' needs. Even worse, they may in the long run damage the communities' interest by interfering with the development of a dependable local capacity to meet those needs.

Swing beds are a makeshift approach to long-term care in which hospitals do not have to meet nursing home standards. Hospitals want to be able to use their acute-care plants for long-term care therapeutic settings. In many cases, this cannot be done, and I find little reason for public acceptance of hospitals performing this function.

Swing beds may also develop an excess capacity that is not needed. For example, Iowa hospitals, which are heavily involved in swing beds, are providing intermediate and private care where there is a very real need for access to medicare skilled care. The result is more duplication of services than the fulfillment of need.

Vladeck's third lesson appears to be that there are important qualitative values offered by swing beds, particularly those relating to being treated in the community. I recognize the important properties that a community-based facility offers, as well as the problems of transfer trauma among the elderly. Nursing homes face these issues as well in their multilevel facilities based in the community. In fact, rural hospitals sometimes serve much larger areas than do community nursing homes and are frequently farther from the patient's home than the nursing home.

What Vladeck has clearly avoided is any kind of realistic comparison between quality of care and life in a swing bed versus that in a nursing home bed. Helen Smits's paper clearly states the case the nursing home industry has been offering in regard to swing beds—that long-term care in nursing homes is superior to care provided in hospital swing beds. The training and expertise of personnel in both types of institutions appear to be one factor but, as Vladeck has failed to understand, the basic component of long-term care is shelter. A long-term care facility is a home that provides along with health care a variety of social amenities that add up, one would hope, to a positive quality of life that most hospital swing beds fail to provide or understand.

Vladeck speaks correctly to the importance of maintaining patients in their home community, not transferring them several times. He cites the swing bed as the way this can be successfully done, but ignores the multilevel nursing home, which has done this successfully for years. He also argues against the current system of levels of care. I think that he would find much support in the nursing home industry for this argument because its leaders call for case mix-based, prospective payment systems. I do not understand how he comes to the conclusion that swing beds are uniquely organized around the needs of patients. My sense is that swing beds' use is clearly tied to reimbursement and decisions about level of care. Rather than a program organized to provide improved services to long-term care patients, it is a program to rescue failing hospitals.

Hospitals have indeed become technologically sophisticated, and their services have gradually excluded those of the elderly who need convalescent and custodial care. But they have done this by choice, and if they have not provided the necessary services to patients awaiting long-term care placement, that is their failure. Do these errors and overly large capital investments in hospital capacity mean supporting the extension of swing beds regardless of need and capacity? I do not think so. I do believe, however, it is necessary to reexamine the need for swing beds and develop the kind of data and analysis that will show how swing beds, rural or urban, can be utilized to meet the service needs of the population.

Comments by Jack W. Owen

THE FIRST lesson Vladeck suggests is that with proper guidance, professional leadership, and regulatory scrutiny hospitals can learn to do reasonably well things they had not done before or at least not done recently. The implication from this lesson is that hospitals are moribund institutions that must be pushed, pulled, or tugged into new services for patients. In reality, hospitals have reacted to societal needs, rules, and reimbursement formulas, rather than to what might be best for treating the patient as a whole. Society was excited about conquering cancer, curing polio, saving heart attack victims, and performing organ transplants and micro-surgery—all noble causes, and most financed quite well. Hospitals were licensed to provide acute care, and without certificate of need, it was an unrestricted license, except for providing long-term care. For instance, in 1962 New Jersey required that a long-term care unit must be physically separated from an acute-care hospital by at least one hundred feet of space in order to be licensed. This was acceptable because that is what society expected and dictated through licensure and the way people, organizations, and government purchased health care insurance or offered health care coverage. Hospitals were just reacting to the marketplace.

The second lesson is that existing capital is less expensive than seeking new capital. With hospitals operating at an 80–85 percent occupancy rate, there were few capital assets available in the acute-care hospital. It was always considered good business to leave a few beds empty in case of a disaster or an epidemic. Since hospitals were paid on a cost reimbursement basis with all costs allocated, the marginal costs of one empty bed were not considered vital to the operation of the institution. Even though hospitals were considered acute-care institutions, the per diem reimbursement system allowed them to provide skilled nursing service beyond the acute-care episode of an illness. Since this is no longer allowed, there has been a drop in length of stay and an increase in empty beds. How to use these community assets in the best possible way is what the swing-bed program is all about.

His third lesson is that people like to receive health services as close to home as possible. One of the reasons the Hill-Burton program was so successful, perhaps too successful, was that every small town wanted its own hospital so that patients did not have to be taken out of their community. There were experiments in the 1950s where programs were established to move patients from small community hospitals to tertiary-care centers and then to a university hospital. One such program was in southwest Michigan, and the reason it was not effective had much to do with the patients' reluctance to be moved from their communities. Not only were the movements of patients to other communities not accepted, the progressive patient-care program met resistance to moving patients just from one floor to another. One of the values of the swing-bed program is that the bed changes; patients do not have to be moved from their community or even from their room.

Institutions should meet the needs of their clients. This is good advice to any organization, and it certainly applies to health care institutions. The biggest problem in carrying out this advice, and Vladeck alludes to it in his paper, is that the institution does not deal directly with the client, but is forced to deal with a third party—government, in the case of medicare—whose major concern is budgetary, not the client's needs. The prospective pricing system has changed the way hospitals operate; it in effect puts a price on a product. Hospitals have reacted by limiting the product to meet the price paid. The problem the patient faces is that the product is not complete. It could almost be compared to selling a refrigerator in today's market without a freezer or ice-making component. Medicare patients do not understand or accept that the price established by the government does not include the time needed to allow them to go home able to care for themselves. Many of those patients do not need long-term chronic care, but need care during a transitional period until they are able to function in a nursing home or a home care setting.

It is on the right track to price services rather than days and to move away from the old cost allocation system. It is going astray to not have the patient or the government pay the price for this transitional care. This is creating a gap in meeting the clients' needs. Hospitals cannot, nor will they, move to provide a service that fills the gap without a method of payment for such a service. The swing-bed programs have shown that the ability to produce is there and the beds needed to meet the needs of the clients are available. What is lacking is the policymakers' willingness to ease the restrictive regulations on the use of those empty beds and a way to pay for the services the clients need.

Contributors

with their affiliations at the time of the conference

Christine E. Bishop
Senior Research Associate, Health Policy Center,
Brandeis University

Raymond Coward
Professor of Social Work, University of Vermont

Steven A. Finkler
Associate Professor, Graduate School of Public Administration,
New York University

Catherine Hawes
Senior Policy Analyst, Research Triangle Institute

John Holahan
Director, Center for Health Policy, Urban Institute

Jacqueline Ann John
Swing-Bed Coordinator, Scott City Hospital

James R. Knickman
Associate Professor, Graduate School of Public Administration,
New York University

Anthony R. Kovner
Program Director, Rural Hospital Program of Extended-Care Services,
New York University

Kenneth Moore
Administrator, Ruidoso Hondo Valley Hospital

Jack W. Owen
Vice-President, American Hospital Association

Stephen Press
Vice-President, American Health Care Association

Hila Richardson
Associate Program Director, Rural Hospital Program
of Extended-Care Services, New York University

139

Peter W. Shaughnessy
Director, Center for Health Services Research, University of Colorado

Robert Schlenker
Senior Associate Director, Health Sciences Center, University of Colorado

Helen L. Smits
Associate Vice-President, Health Center, University of Connecticut

Bruce C. Vladeck
President, United Hospital Fund

Joshua M. Wiener
Senior Fellow, Brookings Institution

Donald A. Wilson
President, Kansas Hospital Association